Life in Recurrence:

Understanding and Living with

Palindromic Rheumatism

D. A. Nyberg

Cover designed with DALL-E and Canva

DEDICATION

To the hope that those primary care physicians who, out of frustration, respond to PR by handing out steroids to help reduce swelling and nothing else, will find the "gumption" to require the specialists to properly diagnosis and treat the PR patients in their care.

FORWARD

When I first experienced the swelling and pain of
PR more than twenty-five years ago and later
diagnosed, by default, with palindromic
rheumatism (PR), I was overwhelmed by questions
that seemed to have no answers. Why was my
body betraying me with sudden, excruciating
flares only to leave me pain-free later? How could
I explain to others a condition that seemed
invisible most of the time? And, perhaps most
hauntingly, what did this mean for my future? Like
so many others living with PR, I felt alone,
confused, and uncertain about the road ahead.

This book was born out of my search for
answers—not just for myself, but for everyone
who shares this journey. As I sought to understand
the complexities of PR, I realized that information
about this condition was scattered and often
inadequate. While there were resources on
autoimmune diseases and arthritis, few focused
on the unique challenges of PR. I wanted more
than just medical definitions—I wanted to

understand how to live fully and confidently despite the uncertainties of this rare condition.

Writing this book became my way of connecting with others, of saying, "You're not alone in this." It's a guide for patients who want to better understand their symptoms, for caregivers looking to support their loved ones, and for anyone trying to navigate the complexities of life with PR. It's also a resource for healthcare providers who may encounter PR in their practice and want to offer more informed care.

In these pages, you'll find lifestyle tips, stories of resilience from people just like you, and insights into the latest research that brings hope for the future. Most importantly, this book is a companion—a reminder that while PR can be isolating, you are part of a community of individuals who understand and share your challenges.

As someone who lives with PR every day, I know how tough it can be. But I also know how empowering it is to arm yourself with knowledge, to connect with others, and to take an active role in your care. This book is for all of us navigating the unpredictable path of PR. Together, we can face its challenges with strength, adaptability, and hope.

Sincerely,

D. A. Nyberg

TABLE OF CONTENTS

INTRODUCTION:

WHAT IS PALINDROMIC RHEUMATISM?

Living with uncertainty can be one of life's greatest challenges, especially when it comes to health. For individuals diagnosed with palindromic rheumatism (PR), the road to understanding their condition is often as unpredictable as the disease itself. PR is a rare and episodic form of inflammatory arthritis characterized by sudden, painful flare-ups in the joints, which disappear just as quickly as they come, leaving little to no lasting damage. This unique "now-you-see-it, now-you-don't" pattern of symptoms makes PR not only challenging to diagnose but also difficult to explain, even to those closest to the person living with it.

The journey through palindromic rheumatism can feel isolating and bewildering. Many people with PR struggle with years of unexplained pain and confusion, often experiencing a range of emotions, from frustration to exhaustion, as they seek answers and relief. The unpredictability of flares adds to the emotional toll, as patients are constantly adapting to periods of intense pain followed by periods of normalcy. Yet, the desire to manage PR and live a full life persists, making knowledge about this condition all the more critical.

Purpose of the Book

This book was written to shed light on the experiences of those living with palindromic rheumatism and to serve as a comprehensive resource for patients, caregivers, healthcare professionals, and anyone else affected by or interested in this unique condition. Here, readers will find detailed information on PR's symptoms, typical and atypical onset patterns, diagnostic challenges, and various approaches to treatment. But beyond medical insights, this book also delves into the daily realities of living with PR—the strategies for coping with flare-ups, the mental and emotional resilience required, and the support systems available.

Whether you are someone newly diagnosed with PR, a loved one supporting someone on this journey, or a healthcare provider looking to deepen your understanding, this book offers a roadmap. It provides medical insights, patient perspectives, and practical tools to help navigate the complexities of PR. As a reader, you will come away with not only a deeper understanding of PR but also an appreciation for the resilience of those who live with it daily.

Structure of the Book

To ensure a complete understanding of palindromic rheumatism, the book is divided into several core sections:

Chapter 1 explores what we currently understand about PR's unique episodic nature, risk factors, and how it is distinguished from other forms of arthritis.

Chapter 2 provides an in-depth look at the symptoms of PR, including both typical and atypical presentations. It also examines how the onset of PR can vary widely from one person to the next, covering cases of sudden and gradual onset, as well as differing initial symptoms.

Chapter 3 addresses the diagnostic process, which can be a challenging road for patients and clinicians alike. The chapter covers tests, imaging, and methods used to differentiate PR from other joint-related conditions, as well as common diagnostic hurdles.

Chapter 4 dives into treatment and management options, including medications, lifestyle adjustments, and complementary therapies. It also includes case studies highlighting various approaches to treatment and their outcomes.

Chapter 5 shifts focus to daily life with PR, including practical advice for managing symptoms, coping with the emotional toll, and balancing daily activities with the unpredictable nature of the disease.

Chapter 6 shares personal stories and perspectives from patients, caregivers, family, and friends. These stories provide a glimpse into the unique challenges and resilience of the PR community.

Chapter 7 explores the latest research on PR, including advances in understanding the immune system's role, new diagnostic tools, and potential future treatments.

Chapter 8 offers a list of resources for PR patients, including support groups, organizations, and educational tools.

Chapter 9 addresses frequently asked questions and common myths about PR, aiming to provide clarity and correct misconceptions.

Finally, the book concludes with reflections on the journey of living with PR, including messages of hope and resilience, and a call to action for continued awareness and advocacy for those affected by this condition.

Who Can Benefit from This Book?

This book is for anyone touched by palindromic rheumatism. Whether you are a patient, a caregiver, a healthcare provider, or simply someone seeking to learn more, you will find information, insight, and empathy within these pages. PR is a condition that deserves recognition and understanding, and this book seeks to give voice to those who live with it.

With knowledge, support, and resources, we hope to empower readers to not only manage PR but to live well in spite of it. Palindromic rheumatism may be unpredictable, but with resilience, community, and care, life with PR can be navigated successfully.

CHAPTER ONE:

UNDERSTANDING PALINDROMIC RHEUMATISM

Palindromic rheumatism (PR) is a rare, episodic form of inflammatory arthritis that presents unique challenges to both patients and medical professionals. Unlike chronic forms of arthritis, which involve continuous joint pain and deterioration, PR is marked by sudden, intense episodes—or "flares"—of pain, swelling, and redness in one or more joints. These flares can last from a few hours to several days, then disappear as quickly as they came, leaving little or no permanent damage to the joints. This seemingly paradoxical pattern of painful symptoms and rapid resolution without lasting effects sets PR apart from other types of arthritis.

In this chapter, we will explore the characteristics of PR, understand who is most affected, and review the known risk factors and potential causes of the condition. Understanding these aspects of PR helps illuminate its nature and prepares patients and healthcare providers for the diagnostic journey.

1. Medical Definition and Characteristics

PR, classified as an inflammatory arthritis, is sometimes considered an early or intermittent form of rheumatoid arthritis (RA), though it also has features that distinguish it from RA and other autoimmune conditions. Key characteristics include:

> **Episodic Nature:** PR presents in flares, with symptoms appearing suddenly and disappearing completely, often within hours or days. Unlike RA, which can lead to chronic joint damage, PR typically leaves no long-term joint deformity or erosion after flares subside.

> **Affected Joints:** PR often targets small joints, particularly in the hands, wrists, and knees, though it can also affect other joints like the shoulders, ankles, and elbows. Each flare can involve different joints, and symptoms may vary in intensity from one episode to another.

Symptom Pattern: Flares often follow a pattern but are notoriously unpredictable. For some, PR may flare up frequently, even weekly, while others experience months between episodes. These symptoms may include joint pain, redness, swelling, warmth, and sometimes fever, making the condition feel more like an acute attack than a chronic illness.

No Long-Term Joint Damage: Unlike many forms of arthritis, PR does not typically cause permanent joint damage, which is a distinguishing factor and often a source of both relief and frustration for patients. Without evidence of erosion, clinicians may struggle to confirm a diagnosis, leading to a cycle of uncertainty for patients.

Understanding these characteristics is crucial because they affect how PR is diagnosed, managed, and lived with day-to-day.

2. Demographics and Prevalence

Palindromic rheumatism is rare, with only an estimated 2.5 out of every 100,000 people affected, and its prevalence varies by region and population. The condition affects both men and women, though women are more likely to be diagnosed, particularly in their mid-20s to early 50s. However, PR can develop in people of any age, including children, and sometimes in elderly populations, making it important for healthcare providers to consider PR as a possibility across all age groups.

The rarity of PR presents unique challenges, as many patients encounter delays in diagnosis or misdiagnosis. As PR lacks the continuous symptomology and visible joint damage that characterizes conditions like RA, physicians and patients alike may dismiss early flares as minor injuries or temporary inflammation. This can lead to prolonged periods of untreated or inadequately managed symptoms for PR patients.

3. Etiology and Risk Factors

The precise cause of palindromic rheumatism remains unknown, although researchers suspect a combination of genetic, environmental, and immunological factors.

Genetic Predisposition: Certain genetic markers, particularly in genes associated with immune function, are thought to increase the likelihood of developing PR. For example, the HLA-DRB1 gene, which has links to RA, has been associated with PR, suggesting shared genetic components between these conditions. However, it's important to note that having these genetic markers does not guarantee PR development.

Immune System Factors: PR is considered an autoimmune condition, where the immune system mistakenly attacks healthy joint tissues, causing inflammation and pain. Studies show that autoantibodies—proteins produced by the immune system that target the body's own cells—are often present in people with PR. The presence of rheumatoid factor (RF) and anti-cyclic citrullinated peptide (anti-CCP) antibodies, commonly seen in RA, can also be found in PR, though not as consistently. This overlap in antibodies complicates distinguishing PR from RA and may contribute to the development of PR symptoms.

Environmental Triggers: Environmental factors may trigger PR flares in susceptible individuals. Common potential triggers include physical stress, infections, and hormonal changes, although the exact mechanism remains unclear. In some cases, flares have been reported after periods of increased physical activity or stress, but these patterns are inconsistent.

Association with Other Autoimmune Conditions: PR often coexists with other autoimmune diseases, such as lupus, Sjögren's syndrome, or even RA, though it remains distinct in its episodic pattern. This association suggests an underlying autoimmune predisposition, where individuals with PR may be more likely to develop other autoimmune conditions, particularly if they carry specific genetic markers.

In summary, while PR shares certain genetic and immunological markers with other autoimmune diseases, its episodic nature and lack of joint damage make it a unique condition. The triggers and mechanisms behind PR remain poorly understood, which is why ongoing research is essential.

4. Typical Progression of Palindromic Rheumatism

PR's course can vary significantly from person to person, making it difficult to predict how the condition will evolve for any given patient. Some experience frequent flares from the beginning, while others may have only a few episodes per year. The lack of a predictable pattern is one of the most challenging aspects of PR.

For some patients, PR may remain episodic and relatively stable for years, with flares becoming less frequent over time. Others, however, may find that their condition gradually shifts toward a chronic inflammatory arthritis, such as rheumatoid arthritis, particularly if they exhibit certain risk factors, like elevated levels of anti-CCP antibodies. Approximately one-third of PR patients develop RA within five years, though this progression is far from guaranteed.

Patients who manage PR successfully often work closely with healthcare providers to monitor their symptoms, test inflammatory markers, and adjust treatments as needed. Early intervention and regular follow-ups can help mitigate the impact of PR and monitor for signs of progression to other forms of arthritis.

Summary

Palindromic rheumatism is a unique, episodic inflammatory condition characterized by painful flares that appear suddenly and disappear without causing lasting joint damage. This feature makes PR distinct from other forms of arthritis, including rheumatoid arthritis, even though the two conditions share some genetic and immunological factors. PR is rare, affecting a small fraction of the population, and presents equally challenging diagnostic and management hurdles due to its unpredictable nature and lack of permanent symptoms.

While the exact cause of PR is unknown, researchers believe a combination of genetic, environmental, and immune factors contribute to its development. The episodic pattern, typical areas of joint involvement, and lack of joint erosion are defining characteristics that shape both the experience of living with PR and the approach to diagnosing and treating it.

In the next chapter, we will delve into the symptoms of PR in greater detail, exploring both typical and atypical presentations and examining how PR's onset can vary widely among patients. Understanding the variability in symptoms and onset is crucial for anyone seeking an accurate diagnosis or a better understanding of this complex condition.

CHAPTER TWO:

SYMPTOMS AND CASE STUDIES

The symptoms of palindromic rheumatism (PR) are as unique as the condition itself, with their episodic, unpredictable nature setting PR apart from other forms of arthritis. A single PR episode, or "flare," can be intense and involve severe joint pain, swelling, and inflammation, only to disappear within a few days, leaving the joint looking and feeling normal again. For patients, these symptoms are often both a source of relief (due to the lack of lasting damage) and frustration, as the pain comes and goes without warning.

In this chapter, we will delve into the typical symptoms of PR, examine atypical presentations, and explore how the condition's onset varies widely among patients. Real-life case studies further illustrate the diversity in PR symptoms, helping to bring this rare condition into clearer focus.

1. Typical Presentation of PR Symptoms

Most people with PR experience a common set of symptoms during flares, which may help distinguish PR from other forms of arthritis.

Joint Pain: Joint pain is often the most immediate and distressing symptom of a PR flare. The pain can be severe, appearing suddenly in one or several joints. The affected joints may be tender to the touch and sensitive to movement, which can limit a person's mobility during a flare.

Swelling and Redness: Flares often cause noticeable swelling around the joint, accompanied by redness and a warm sensation. This inflammation is a sign of the immune system's activity within the joint. Swelling may make the joint appear larger than usual, which can be alarming for patients experiencing it for the first time.

Joint Involvement: PR often targets the small joints in the hands and wrists, though it can affect any joint in the body, including the knees, ankles, shoulders, and elbows. Joint involvement during flares is unpredictable, with different joints affected from one episode to the next.

Symptom Duration: The duration of a flare can vary, lasting anywhere from a few hours to several days. Some patients experience flares that start in the evening and resolve by morning, while others may have episodes that persist for days. Between flares, patients may experience no symptoms and feel completely well.

Systemic Symptoms: In addition to joint pain, some patients may experience low-grade fevers, fatigue, and a general sense of malaise during flares. These systemic symptoms are less common but can add to the physical and emotional toll of the condition.

These typical symptoms form a recognizable pattern that, over time, helps patients and their healthcare providers identify PR. However, the variability in symptoms from one flare to the next can make early diagnosis challenging.

2. Atypical Cases of PR

While most patients with PR experience symptoms in a somewhat predictable pattern, there are also atypical presentations that can complicate diagnosis.

Unusual Joint Patterns: In rare cases, PR can affect the same joint repeatedly or only a single joint throughout the course of the disease, which is atypical for PR but may occur. Some patients may experience flares that affect large joints only, like the hips or shoulders, which is less common than the involvement of small joints.

Mild or Subtle Flares: Some patients report flares that are mild or even subclinical, meaning that inflammation occurs but causes minimal pain or swelling. In these cases, laboratory markers of inflammation may rise, but physical symptoms are minimal, leading to diagnostic confusion.

Extended Flares with Mild Symptoms: Another atypical pattern involves extended flares with relatively mild symptoms, where patients experience prolonged episodes of discomfort that are more chronic in nature. These episodes may cause lingering soreness or stiffness in affected joints, creating confusion with conditions like osteoarthritis.

Systemic Involvement Beyond Joints: While rare, some patients with PR report symptoms outside of the joints, such as swelling of soft tissues or even signs of inflammation in areas like tendons or muscles. Though these cases are uncommon, they demonstrate the range of experiences possible within PR.

Atypical cases emphasize the need for healthcare providers to consider PR even when symptoms deviate from the classical pattern, as early diagnosis and management can improve quality of life for patients.

3. Onset of Palindromic Rheumatism

The onset of PR is another area where variation is common, with different patients reporting different experiences when symptoms first appear.

Typical Onset Patterns:

Gradual Onset: Some patients experience a gradual onset, where symptoms begin mildly, with occasional joint pain or discomfort that worsens over time. This can make early symptoms easy to overlook or dismiss as joint strain or mild arthritis.

Sudden Onset: For others, PR begins suddenly with a severe, unexplained flare affecting one or more joints. This abrupt onset can mimic an acute injury or infection, often leading patients to seek immediate medical care.

Differing Onset Processes:

Flare-Based Onset: Many PR patients first notice the condition through isolated flares that appear and resolve unpredictably. Initially, these flares may be spread out over months, giving a deceptive impression of infrequent or mi nor joint issues.

Subclinical Onset: In some cases, PR onset is subtle, with mild inflammatory activity occurring without noticeable symptoms. Blood tests may reveal elevated inflammatory markers, but patients do not initially experience significant joint pain or swelling.

Onset with Other Autoimmune Conditions: Some individuals develop PR alongside another autoimmune disease, such as lupus or Sjögren's syndrome. The coexistence of these conditions can obscure PR's distinct episodic nature, leading to potential delays in identifying PR as a separate condition.

Age-Related Onset Differences: Onset can also vary by age. Younger patients, for example, may experience more sudden and intense flares, while older patients may have a slower, more insidious onset.

The diversity in PR's onset highlights why many patients experience delayed or uncertain diagnoses. Recognizing these patterns and understanding their variability is essential for anyone managing or diagnosing PR.

4. Case Studies of PR Patients

To illustrate the range of PR symptoms and onset patterns, the following case studies provide real-life examples of how the condition manifests and evolves over time. These stories capture the diversity of PR and demonstrate the importance of personalized care.

Case Study 1: Sarah's Flare-Based Onset and Unpredictable Pattern

Background: Sarah, a 35-year-old teacher, began experiencing unexplained joint pain in her hands and knees. The pain would come on suddenly and resolve within a day, leaving her joint feeling entirely normal.

Symptoms: Initially, Sarah's flares were mild and infrequent, but over time, they increased in frequency, affecting different joints with varying intensity. She struggled to convey the severity of her symptoms to her doctor, as each flare would resolve before she could see a specialist.

Outcome: Sarah was eventually diagnosed with PR after keeping a symptom diary, which documented her flares and helped her rheumatologist identify a pattern.

Case Study 2: James's Sudden, Severe Onset

Background: James, a 42-year-old construction worker, developed PR suddenly with intense pain in his wrists and shoulders. The pain was so severe that he initially suspected a serious injury, although imaging showed no joint damage.

Symptoms: His flares would last several days, causing significant inflammation, but would resolve completely between episodes. The sudden onset and severity led to multiple medical evaluations before PR was identified.

Outcome: James's diagnosis enabled him to begin treatment, which helped manage his symptoms and reduced the intensity of his flares.

Case Study 3: Maria's Mild, Subclinical Onset

Background: Maria, a 50-year-old office worker, experienced subtle symptoms over the course of a year, with occasional joint stiffness and mild swelling. Her primary care physician initially attributed her symptoms to osteoarthritis.

Symptoms: After a particularly intense flare in her knee, she underwent further testing that revealed inflammatory markers consistent with PR.

Outcome: Maria's story highlights the challenges of identifying PR in cases with mild or atypical symptoms.

Each of these cases demonstrates the diverse presentation of PR and underscores the importance of recognizing atypical symptoms and onset patterns. For patients and clinicians alike, understanding this variability is key to achieving timely diagnosis and effective management.

Summary

The symptoms of palindromic rheumatism are as unpredictable as the disease itself. PR's episodic flares, which can range from mild to severe, may appear suddenly and affect different joints with each episode. While typical symptoms include joint pain, swelling, and redness, atypical presentations remind us that PR is a variable condition that doesn't always fit a predictable mold.

Understanding the onset of PR is equally important. Patients may experience symptoms that come on suddenly or gradually, with some people seeing prolonged intervals between flares, while others experience frequent episodes. Real-life case studies illustrate these differences and highlight the importance of patient awareness and physician vigilance in achieving an accurate diagnosis.

In the next chapter, we will explore the diagnostic process for PR, examining the tests, imaging techniques, and challenges associated with diagnosing this rare and often misunderstood condition. By understanding the diagnostic pathway, patients and providers can work together to establish an effective treatment plan and improve quality of life.

CHAPTER THREE:

DIAGNOSIS OF PALINDROMIC RHEUMATISM

Diagnosing palindromic rheumatism (PR) is often a complex process. The episodic nature of PR, with flares that disappear and leave no lasting joint damage, makes it hard to identify and even harder to confirm. This is why patients frequently undergo a lengthy diagnostic journey, sometimes facing misdiagnoses or inconclusive results before PR is considered. In this chapter, we will walk through the diagnostic steps for PR, covering initial assessments, laboratory tests, imaging, and differential diagnoses.

Understanding the diagnostic process is essential for both patients and healthcare providers, as timely diagnosis allows for more effective management and monitoring of PR symptoms, potentially slowing or preventing the progression to more chronic forms of arthritis.

1. The Diagnostic Process

The diagnosis of PR begins with a thorough assessment of the patient's medical history, a physical examination, and documentation of symptom patterns. Because PR symptoms are episodic, it is often challenging to capture flare symptoms directly during a clinical visit, making patient history and self-reported symptom patterns crucial for diagnosis.

Initial Assessment: A healthcare provider begins by asking about the nature, frequency, and duration of the patient's symptoms. Patients with PR often report sudden-onset joint pain, swelling, and redness that resolves within hours to days. Identifying a pattern of such episodic symptoms is key to distinguishing PR from other conditions that cause persistent or progressive joint pain.

Symptom Pattern Documentation: Patients are often encouraged to keep a symptom diary, documenting the timing, location, and severity of each flare. This record can provide valuable insights into the episodic nature of PR, as well as any triggers, such as stress, physical exertion, or hormonal changes, that might precipitate flares.

Physical Examination: During a clinical visit, the physician will examine any affected joints if the patient is currently experiencing a flare. However, because PR flares are often short-lived, patients may be asymptomatic during the appointment. If there is no active flare, the physical examination may reveal little to no signs of joint damage or inflammation, which differentiates PR from conditions like rheumatoid arthritis (RA), where chronic inflammation leads to visible joint damage over time.

The initial assessment is crucial in establishing a pattern that points to PR. However, due to the condition's rarity, further testing is often needed to confirm the diagnosis and rule out other conditions.

2. Diagnostic Tests and Markers

After the initial assessment, physicians may order specific laboratory tests and imaging studies to identify inflammatory markers, detect autoantibodies, and rule out other conditions. Although there are no definitive tests for PR, the following tests can support the diagnosis.

Laboratory Tests:

> **Rheumatoid Factor (RF):** RF is an antibody commonly associated with RA. Although it is not present in all cases of PR, about 30-50% of PR patients test positive for RF. However, a positive RF test alone is not diagnostic, as RF can also be elevated in other autoimmune diseases and even in healthy individuals.

> **Anti-Cyclic Citrullinated Peptide (Anti-CCP) Antibodies:** Anti-CCP is another antibody commonly found in RA and can be present in some PR patients, particularly those at risk of progressing to RA. The presence of anti-CCP antibodies is associated with more severe and frequent flares in PR, and about

20-40% of PR patients test positive for this antibody.

Antinuclear Antibodies (ANA): ANA testing screens for the presence of autoantibodies often found in autoimmune diseases like lupus. Some PR patients may test positive for ANA, though this test is not specific to PR and cannot alone confirm a diagnosis.

Inflammatory Markers: Blood tests measuring markers of inflammation, such as erythrocyte sedimentation rate (ESR) and C-reactive protein (CRP), are typically elevated during PR flares. If tested during an active flare, these markers can indicate an inflammatory process, but in the absence of a flare, they may return to normal, making it hard to rely on inflammatory markers alone.

Imaging Techniques:

X-Rays: X-rays of the affected joints are typically normal in PR patients, as the disease does not cause permanent joint damage. However, if there is any suspicion of RA or another chronic arthritis, X-rays can help rule out visible joint erosion.

Ultrasound and MRI: In some cases, ultrasound or MRI may reveal temporary inflammation or fluid in the joints, even in the absence of visible joint damage. These imaging techniques can be particularly useful in capturing subtle changes during a flare, as they can detect early signs of synovitis (inflammation of the joint lining) and effusion (fluid accumulation) in the joints. MRIs are especially helpful for visualizing soft tissue inflammation, which may be undetectable by X-ray.

These tests, while informative, are not specific enough to diagnose PR on their own. Together with the patient's medical history and symptom pattern, however, they can help provide strong evidence of PR when other conditions are ruled out.

3. Differential Diagnosis

Because PR's symptoms overlap with those of other joint-related and autoimmune conditions, differential diagnosis is essential. Healthcare providers must carefully differentiate PR from other diseases that cause joint pain, swelling, and inflammation.

Rheumatoid Arthritis (RA): RA is one of the most commonly mistaken conditions for PR due to the presence of joint pain, swelling, and autoantibodies like RF and anti-CCP. However, RA is characterized by persistent inflammation and progressive joint damage, whereas PR flares are transient, leaving no long-term joint damage. Additionally, RA usually affects joints symmetrically, while PR does not follow a fixed pattern.

Lupus and Other Autoimmune Conditions: Systemic lupus erythematosus (SLE) and other autoimmune conditions like Sjögren's syndrome can present with joint pain, swelling, and positive ANA tests, similar to PR. However, these conditions often have systemic symptoms beyond joint involvement, such as skin rashes, kidney involvement, and specific laboratory markers unique to each disease.

Gout and Pseudogout: Gout and pseudogout are forms of inflammatory arthritis that cause sudden, severe pain in the joints, often affecting the big toe or knee. Unlike PR, these conditions are caused by crystal deposits in the joints (uric acid in gout and calcium pyrophosphate in pseudogout), which can be confirmed through joint fluid analysis and testing for uric acid levels.

Reactive Arthritis: Reactive arthritis, which can occur following an infection, shares some symptoms with PR, including joint pain and swelling. However, reactive arthritis is often accompanied by other symptoms, such as eye inflammation, urethritis, or skin lesions, which are not characteristic of PR.

Osteoarthritis (OA): OA is a degenerative joint disease commonly associated with aging and wear-and-tear of the joints. Unlike PR, which presents with inflammatory flares, OA is marked by chronic joint pain, stiffness, and cartilage breakdown, typically affecting weight-bearing joints and showing joint changes on X-rays.

The process of ruling out these conditions requires careful consideration and sometimes repeated testing, especially given PR's episodic nature. This diagnostic complexity can lead to delays, making it essential for both patients and clinicians to understand the distinct features of PR.

4. Challenges in Diagnosing PR

Diagnosing PR is challenging for both patients and healthcare providers due to several factors:

Episodic Nature of Symptoms: PR flares are temporary and may resolve before a patient can seek medical evaluation, leading some providers to misinterpret the condition as psychosomatic or minor. Without visible joint damage, it can be difficult to verify a history of flares.

Lack of Definitive Testing: Unlike other forms of arthritis, there are no specific tests that conclusively diagnose PR. Instead, diagnosis relies on a combination of patient history, symptom pattern, and exclusion of other conditions.

Limited Awareness: PR is a rare condition, and its symptoms may be mistaken for those of more common types of arthritis. Patients may experience delays in diagnosis if healthcare providers are unfamiliar with PR or if the patient's symptom pattern does not initially align with PR.

Overlap with Other Autoimmune Diseases: Some patients with PR may have overlapping autoimmune conditions, complicating the diagnostic process. Patients with positive tests for RF, anti-CCP, or ANA may be suspected of having RA or lupus, and distinguishing between these conditions is critical to ensure accurate diagnosis and treatment.

Understanding these challenges can empower patients to advocate for themselves in the diagnostic process and help healthcare providers consider PR even when it presents atypically.

Summary

Diagnosing palindromic rheumatism requires a careful balance of clinical observation, laboratory testing, and exclusion of other conditions. The episodic nature of PR, combined with the lack of specific diagnostic tests, makes diagnosis a challenge for both patients and healthcare providers. Laboratory markers like RF and anti-CCP, along with imaging techniques such as ultrasound and MRI, can provide helpful clues, especially during active flares. However, since PR shares symptoms with several other forms of arthritis and autoimmune diseases, a detailed patient history and differential diagnosis are key.

For patients, understanding the complexities of PR diagnosis can empower them to document their symptoms, communicate effectively with healthcare providers, and seek specialists if necessary. With a clearer diagnosis, patients can begin appropriate treatment, which can improve symptom management and overall quality of life.

In the next chapter, we will explore treatment and management options for PR, from medications to lifestyle changes and complementary therapies. By understanding the available treatments, patients and their providers can work together to reduce the impact of PR and enhance day-to-day well-being.

CHAPTER FOUR:

TREATMENT AND MANAGEMENT OPTIONS

Living with palindromic rheumatism (PR) involves managing unpredictable flares of joint pain and inflammation. Although PR currently has no cure, various treatments can help reduce flare frequency, minimize symptoms, and improve overall quality of life. Treatment approaches for PR range from pharmaceutical options to complementary therapies and lifestyle modifications. This chapter examines each of these approaches, providing a comprehensive overview of how patients and healthcare providers can work together to manage PR effectively.

Through the treatment options outlined here, patients can explore ways to regain a sense of control over their condition, despite its episodic and unpredictable nature.

1. Medications for PR

Medication is often the cornerstone of managing PR, as it can help reduce the intensity and frequency of flares. While there are no treatments specifically approved for PR, medications used to treat rheumatoid arthritis (RA) and other autoimmune conditions can be effective.

Nonsteroidal Anti-Inflammatory Drugs (NSAIDs):

> NSAIDs, such as ibuprofen and naproxen, are frequently used during flares to relieve pain and reduce inflammation. They are often the first line of treatment due to their effectiveness in reducing the immediate discomfort associated with flares.

> Advantages and Limitations: NSAIDs provide quick relief but are not suitable for long-term daily use due to potential side effects, such as gastrointestinal issues and increased cardiovascular risk. Patients are typically advised to use NSAIDs as needed, rather than daily, unless under medical supervision.

Corticosteroids:

> Corticosteroids, like prednisone, are powerful anti-inflammatory medications that can quickly alleviate the symptoms of PR flares. They are generally prescribed in short courses to manage severe flares.

> Advantages and Limitations: While effective, corticosteroids are not recommended for long-term use due to risks of side effects, such as weight gain, osteoporosis, and increased infection risk. Physicians may prescribe a short course of corticosteroids during intense flares to help patients regain mobility and reduce pain swiftly.

Disease-Modifying Antirheumatic Drugs (DMARDs):

> DMARDs, particularly hydroxychloroquine, are commonly prescribed to reduce flare frequency and severity. Hydroxychloroquine is frequently used in PR and has shown effectiveness in controlling symptoms over time, with fewer side effects compared to other DMARDs.

Advantages and Limitations: DMARDs can reduce inflammation and may help prevent the progression of PR to other forms of arthritis, such as RA. However, they may take weeks or months to show full effects, requiring patience. Regular monitoring is essential, especially with drugs like methotrexate, due to potential side effects on the liver and immune system.

Biologic Agents:

Although not commonly used in PR, biologic agents—like TNF inhibitors and interleukin inhibitors—are sometimes prescribed in cases where PR symptoms are severe or resistant to other treatments. Biologics are more commonly associated with RA but may benefit PR patients with chronic or aggressive symptoms.

Advantages and Limitations: Biologics are highly effective for inflammation but come with a higher cost and require regular injections or infusions. They also carry a risk of serious side effects, including increased susceptibility to infections.

The choice of medication depends on individual symptoms, flare frequency, and patient tolerance. Many PR patients find that a combination of NSAIDs and a DMARD like hydroxychloroquine offers effective symptom management with minimal side effects.

2. Alternative and Complementary Treatments

In addition to conventional medications, many PR patients find relief through complementary therapies. While not replacements for medical treatment, these therapies can support well-being and symptom management.

Physical Therapy and Occupational Therapy:

> Physical therapy helps improve joint mobility, strengthen muscles, and reduce stiffness, which can benefit patients both during and between flares. Occupational therapists can provide tools and strategies to reduce joint strain in daily activities.

> Advantages and Limitations: Physical and occupational therapies are non-invasive and improve quality of life without medication-

related side effects. However, the benefits are usually limited to managing symptoms rather than preventing flares.

Acupuncture:

Acupuncture, a traditional Chinese medicine practice, may provide pain relief for some PR patients. By inserting fine needles into specific points on the body, acupuncture aims to stimulate energy flow and reduce inflammation.

Advantages and Limitations: While many patients report pain relief, scientific evidence on acupuncture's effectiveness for PR is limited. Results can vary widely, and some may need multiple sessions to experience benefits.

Dietary Modifications and Supplements:

Some patients explore dietary changes to help reduce inflammation and manage flares. Anti-inflammatory diets rich in omega-3 fatty acids, antioxidants, and whole foods may help, while avoiding processed foods and refined sugars. Supplements like turmeric, fish oil, and vitamin D are also commonly used.

Advantages and Limitations: While dietary changes can support overall health and possibly reduce inflammation, they are not a standalone treatment for PR. Patients are encouraged to consult healthcare providers before starting supplements, as some may interact with medications.

Mindfulness and Stress-Reduction Techniques:

Mindfulness practices, such as meditation, yoga, and breathing exercises, help reduce stress, which can act as a flare trigger for some PR patients. Practicing mindfulness regularly can enhance mental resilience and improve pain perception.

Advantages and Limitations: These techniques support mental health and are generally safe, though they may not directly reduce inflammation. Regular practice is essential to see benefits.

Integrating complementary treatments with medical therapies can offer a well-rounded approach to managing PR. However, patients should discuss these options with their healthcare provider to ensure safety and compatibility with prescribed medications.

3. Lifestyle Adjustments

Adjusting lifestyle habits can play a significant role in managing PR. These adjustments help patients cope with the condition's unpredictable nature and maintain a high quality of life.

Managing Physical Activity:

> Staying active is essential for joint health, but overexertion can trigger PR flares. Low-impact exercises like swimming, walking, and cycling can help improve flexibility, strength, and cardiovascular health without stressing the joints.

> Practical Tips: Patients are encouraged to balance activity and rest. Tracking symptoms can help identify when certain

activities or levels of intensity might trigger flares.

Sleep and Rest:

Quality sleep is vital for immune health and recovery. PR patients may need more rest during or after flares to help their bodies recuperate.

Practical Tips: Establishing a regular sleep schedule and using relaxation techniques before bed can improve sleep quality. Patients are also encouraged to rest between flares to avoid burnout.

Using Assistive Devices:

Assistive devices, such as joint supports, braces, and ergonomic tools, can help reduce joint strain during daily tasks. Simple tools, like jar openers or cushioned mats, can make a significant difference in comfort and joint protection.

Practical Tips: Occupational therapists can recommend devices based on individual needs, helping patients navigate daily activities without aggravating their joints.

Maintaining a Healthy Diet:

Eating a balanced, nutrient-rich diet can help support immune function and reduce inflammation. An anti-inflammatory diet that includes fruits, vegetables, whole grains, lean proteins, and healthy fats is often recommended.

Practical Tips: Reducing processed foods, sugary drinks, and red meat may help lower inflammation levels. Drinking adequate water and staying hydrated also aids in joint health.

Mental Health and Social Support:

The unpredictable nature of PR can take a toll on mental well-being. Patients are encouraged to seek support through therapy, support groups, or online communities, where they can connect with others who understand the challenges of living with PR.

Practical Tips: Building a support network of family, friends, and healthcare professionals provides emotional strength. Cognitive-behavioral therapy (CBT) and mindfulness meditation are helpful strategies for managing anxiety related to the unpredictability of PR.

By making lifestyle adjustments, patients can improve their resilience, reduce triggers, and feel more empowered in managing their PR.

4. Case Studies of Treatment Approaches

To illustrate the diversity of treatment experiences, the following case studies highlight different approaches to managing PR symptoms.

Case Study 1: Lisa's Combination of Medication and Lifestyle Changes

Background: Lisa, a 40-year-old marketing executive, began experiencing PR flares affecting her hands and knees. She started with NSAIDs during flares but found them insufficient for longer-term relief.

Treatment Approach: Lisa's rheumatologist prescribed hydroxychloroquine as a long-term treatment and NSAIDs as needed for flares. She also implemented lifestyle changes, such as adopting an anti-inflammatory diet and practicing yoga.

Outcome: With this combination, Lisa experienced fewer flares, and her overall pain was reduced. She reports feeling more in control of her symptoms and is able to stay active in her job and personal life.

Case Study 2: David's Use of Physical Therapy and Stress Management

Background: David, a 55-year-old teacher, initially avoided medication, hoping his PR symptoms would subside. However, his flares persisted, affecting his knees and shoulders.

Treatment Approach: After consulting a physical therapist, David began a gentle exercise routine to improve joint stability and flexibility. He also practiced mindfulness meditation to help manage stress, which he identified as a flare trigger.

Outcome: Although David occasionally requires NSAIDs, his physical therapy routine and mindfulness practice have significantly reduced his flare frequency, allowing him to continue teaching with minimal disruption.

Case Study 3: Maria's Use of Biologics for Severe PR Symptoms

Background: Maria, a 47-year-old artist, experienced frequent and intense flares, which limited her ability to work and caused her significant pain.

Treatment Approach: After trying NSAIDs and hydroxychloroquine with limited success, Maria's rheumatologist prescribed a biologic medication. Maria also incorporated acupuncture and dietary changes into her routine.

Outcome: Since starting the biologic, Maria has seen a marked reduction in the severity and frequency of her flares. The combination of medical and complementary treatments has helped her regain her ability to work and manage her symptoms more effectively.

Each of these case studies demonstrates how PR patients can benefit from personalized treatment plans that incorporate medications, lifestyle changes, and complementary therapies.

Summary

Treating and managing palindromic rheumatism requires a multi-faceted approach tailored to each patient's unique symptoms and lifestyle. Medications such as NSAIDs, corticosteroids, DMARDs, and, in severe cases, biologics are commonly used to control inflammation and reduce flare frequency. Complementary treatments, such as physical therapy, acupuncture, dietary modifications, and mindfulness practices, provide additional support for symptom management and overall well-being.

Lifestyle adjustments, including exercise, sleep hygiene, assistive devices, and mental health support, empower patients to live with greater ease and resilience. Through a combination of these treatments and adjustments, PR patients can take an active role in managing their condition and improving their quality of life.

In the next chapter, we will discuss the daily realities of living with PR, exploring practical advice, emotional coping strategies, and ways to build resilience in the face of an unpredictable illness.

CHAPTER FIVE:

LIVING WITH PALINDROMIC RHEUMATISM

Living with palindromic rheumatism (PR) means adapting to an unpredictable cycle of joint pain and inflammation that can affect nearly every aspect of daily life. The intermittent nature of PR creates unique challenges, as individuals often find themselves alternating between painful flare-ups and symptom-free periods. This inconsistency makes it difficult for PR patients to plan their daily activities, manage their responsibilities, and maintain relationships. It also affects emotional well-being, as the unpredictable onset of flares can lead to anxiety, frustration, and even social isolation.

In this chapter, we will explore strategies for managing day-to-day life with PR, including ways to cope with physical symptoms, approaches to maintaining mental health, and practical tips for balancing activity and rest. By understanding and implementing these strategies, PR patients can enhance their quality of life and better navigate the complexities of this condition.

1. The Emotional and Mental Health Impact of PR

The emotional impact of PR is often as significant as the physical symptoms, if not more so. Coping with sudden, recurring joint pain and the unpredictability of flares can lead to stress, anxiety, and depression. It is common for PR patients to feel frustrated, isolated, or misunderstood, as their condition is not always apparent to others. Addressing mental health needs is essential for overall well-being.

Coping with Uncertainty:

> The unpredictable nature of PR means patients never know when a flare may occur, making it difficult to plan ahead. This uncertainty can lead to anxiety, especially in social or work settings where sudden pain can disrupt routines. To manage uncertainty, patients can focus on what they can control—such as self-care routines, preparing flare kits, and having support systems in place.

Managing Anxiety and Depression:

Anxiety and depression are common among individuals with chronic conditions like PR. Practicing mindfulness techniques, such as meditation or deep breathing exercises, can help reduce anxiety by grounding patients in the present moment. Cognitive behavioral therapy (CBT) can also be an effective tool in addressing negative thought patterns associated with pain and uncertainty.

Building Resilience:

Building resilience involves developing mental and emotional strength to cope with the highs and lows of PR. Patients can focus on personal goals, cultivate hobbies, and seek support through friends, family, or support groups to build resilience. Resilience is not about ignoring the challenges but finding ways to navigate them with hope and purpose.

Seeking Professional Help:

> Speaking with a mental health professional, such as a therapist or counselor, can help PR patients manage the emotional toll of the disease. Therapy can provide coping strategies, emotional validation, and a safe space to express frustrations. Support groups, both in-person and online, also offer community and shared experiences that reduce feelings of isolation.

By acknowledging and addressing the emotional aspects of PR, patients can maintain better mental health, which in turn supports their physical well-being.

2. Day-to-Day Management of Symptoms

Effectively managing PR symptoms day-to-day involves learning how to handle flares, balance activity and rest, and use tools or modifications to reduce strain on affected joints. While each individual's experience with PR may vary, adopting these strategies can make a significant difference in managing symptoms.

Managing Pain and Fatigue During Flares:

Pain Relief Techniques: During a flare, pain can be intense, making it difficult to move or focus. Applying heat or cold packs to inflamed joints can offer relief—heat can ease stiffness, while cold can reduce swelling and numb pain. Over-the-counter medications, such as NSAIDs, can also provide temporary relief.

Gentle Stretching and Movement: Light stretching or gentle movement, as tolerated, can help maintain joint mobility without placing excessive strain on the affected area. This is especially helpful if certain joints become stiff during flares.

Rest and Recovery: Resting during and after a flare allows the body to recover and reduce inflammation. Patients should listen to their bodies and prioritize rest over exertion during painful episodes.

Balancing Activity and Rest:

Pacing Activities: Pacing involves breaking tasks into smaller steps and taking breaks to avoid overexertion. PR patients often find it helpful to alternate between active periods and rest, especially during longer tasks, to prevent flares triggered by excessive activity.

Planning Ahead: Planning tasks around flare patterns or scheduling challenging activities during symptom-free periods can help patients manage responsibilities more effectively. For instance, a patient might reserve more demanding activities for the morning if they know their flares typically occur in the afternoon.

Setting Boundaries: Learning to say "no" or delegate tasks can help PR patients conserve energy and avoid activities that may exacerbate symptoms. Setting boundaries is particularly useful for preventing exhaustion, both physically and mentally.

Using Assistive Devices:

Assistive devices, such as ergonomic kitchen tools, jar openers, walking aids, and joint braces, can reduce strain on the joints and make daily activities easier. Occupational therapists can recommend specific tools based on the patient's needs and lifestyle, offering tailored solutions to support independence.

These day-to-day management strategies can improve comfort and mobility for PR patients, helping them stay active without triggering additional flares.

3. Lifestyle Adjustments

Incorporating certain lifestyle adjustments can enhance symptom management, reduce flare frequency, and support overall health. These adjustments include focusing on diet, exercise, sleep, and hydration.

Importance of Diet:

> Many PR patients find that dietary choices influence their symptoms. An anti-inflammatory diet, which includes fruits, vegetables, whole grains, lean proteins, and

healthy fats (like omega-3s), may help reduce overall inflammation. Avoiding processed foods, sugary drinks, and red meat can also support better health and potentially decrease flare severity.

Supplements: Some patients use supplements like turmeric, omega-3 fish oil, or vitamin D to support joint health. However, it is important to consult a healthcare provider before starting any supplements, as they may interact with medications.

Exercise and Physical Activity:

Regular exercise, tailored to the patient's abilities and flare patterns, can improve joint strength, flexibility, and cardiovascular health. Low-impact exercises, such as swimming, cycling, and walking, are generally recommended for PR patients, as they are gentle on the joints.

Stretching and Range-of-Motion Exercises: Regular stretching and range-of-motion exercises can help maintain joint mobility and reduce stiffness. Practicing these exercises daily, even between flares, helps keep the joints flexible and minimizes discomfort.

Sleep and Rest:

Adequate sleep is essential for immune health and recovery, and PR patients often require extra rest during flares. Establishing a consistent sleep routine, including a calm bedtime environment and limiting screen time before bed, can improve sleep quality.

Listening to the Body's Signals: PR patients should pay attention to signs of fatigue, especially after a flare, and allow themselves time to rest without guilt. This helps ensure that the body has time to recover and reduce inflammation effectively.

Staying Hydrated:

Drinking adequate water supports joint health and overall bodily function. Staying hydrated is especially important for PR patients, as dehydration can sometimes exacerbate joint pain.

By integrating these lifestyle adjustments into their routines, PR patients can support their health and potentially reduce flare frequency or severity.

4. Practical Tips for Social and Professional Life

PR's unpredictability can impact a patient's social and professional life, making it challenging to maintain relationships and work commitments. However, there are practical strategies that PR patients can adopt to stay engaged and manage their responsibilities effectively.

Communicating Needs:

> Open communication with family, friends, and colleagues about PR and its impact can foster understanding and reduce feelings of isolation. Being honest about flare-ups and any necessary limitations allows others to support the patient more effectively.

> Educating Others: PR is often not well-understood by the general public, so

explaining the condition and how it differs from other forms of arthritis can help loved ones and coworkers better appreciate its challenges.

Adapting the Work Environment:

PR patients may need to make adjustments to their work environments to avoid flare triggers. For example, an ergonomic chair, supportive desk setup, or assistive devices can reduce strain. Remote work options and flexible hours, where possible, provide additional support for managing flares.

Requesting Accommodations: Many workplaces offer accommodations for employees with chronic conditions. Patients may benefit from requesting modifications, such as short breaks throughout the day, to manage symptoms more effectively.

Maintaining Social Connections:

Although PR's unpredictability can make it hard to attend social events, maintaining social connections is important for emotional well-being. Patients can plan gatherings during symptom-free periods or host events at home to create a comfortable, flare-friendly environment.

Using Virtual Options: Online meetups and video calls are helpful alternatives for maintaining social connections when attending in-person events is challenging. Virtual connections can also provide a sense of community, especially during difficult flare periods.

Balancing social and professional life with PR requires flexibility, patience, and honest communication. By adapting routines and utilizing support systems, PR patients can continue to engage in meaningful relationships and activities.

Summary

Living with palindromic rheumatism is a complex journey that involves adapting to an unpredictable condition that impacts physical, emotional, and social aspects of life. Day-to-day management strategies, such as pacing, using assistive devices, and practicing gentle exercise, empower PR patients to stay active and independent. Addressing the emotional toll of PR is equally important, and tools like mindfulness, therapy, and support groups can significantly improve mental health.

Lifestyle adjustments, including a balanced diet, regular exercise, quality sleep, and adequate hydration, provide a solid foundation for managing symptoms and promoting overall health. Finally, practical strategies for work and social life help patients maintain connections and responsibilities without overextending themselves. With these approaches, PR patients can lead fulfilling lives, despite the challenges posed by their condition.

In the next chapter, we will explore patient and caregiver stories that offer personal insights into living with PR, showing the resilience and adaptability that many individuals develop to navigate the ups and downs of this unique condition.

CHAPTER SIX:

PATIENT AND CAREGIVER STORIES

Living with palindromic rheumatism (PR) is a journey that requires resilience, patience, and adaptability—not only from the patients themselves but also from the family members, friends, and caregivers who support them. Every PR journey is unique, shaped by the unpredictable nature of the condition and the emotional and physical demands it places on those affected. This chapter offers real-life stories and insights from PR patients, caregivers, and loved ones, illustrating the strength and hope that drive them forward.

Through these stories, we gain a closer look at how people navigate life with PR, from coping with sudden flares to maintaining relationships and finding purpose amid challenges. By sharing these experiences, we hope to provide encouragement, empathy, and understanding to others on similar journeys.

1. Perspectives from Patients

The voices of PR patients reveal the personal toll of living with a condition that is not only physically painful but often misunderstood by others. These stories highlight the strategies patients use to adapt and thrive despite the limitations PR imposes.

Case Study 1: Sarah's Story of Resilience and Adaptation

> Background: Sarah, a 35-year-old teacher, was diagnosed with PR five years ago after experiencing recurrent episodes of intense joint pain in her hands, wrists, and knees. She describes her early days of diagnosis as a period filled with uncertainty and frustration, as she struggled to understand her symptoms and communicate her needs to her loved ones and colleagues.

> Living with Flares: Sarah recounts the daily challenges of dealing with unpredictable flares. She has learned to keep a "flare kit" with pain relief options, heating pads, and a journal to track symptoms. Through trial and error, she's discovered that pacing her

activities and planning for rest after busy days helps her prevent flares.

Emotional Journey: Sarah candidly shares the emotional journey of living with PR, including moments of despair and the eventual acceptance of her limitations. She found support through online communities and decided to start a blog, where she shares her journey and offers practical advice to other PR patients.

Message to Others: "PR taught me to take things one day at a time and celebrate small victories. Even though I can't predict the flares, I can choose how to respond to them. Finding a community that understands has been a lifeline, reminding me that I'm not alone in this."

Case Study 2: David's Approach to Mindful Living

Background: David, a 50-year-old therapist, was diagnosed with PR seven years ago after experiencing intermittent flares in his knees, shoulders, and hands. His journey with PR has been deeply influenced by his profession, as he often turns to mindfulness and emotional resilience practices to manage his symptoms.

Daily Coping Techniques: David practices mindfulness meditation daily, which he credits with helping him stay calm during flares. He also uses cognitive behavioral therapy (CBT) techniques to manage the anxiety that accompanies the uncertainty of PR.

Impact on Relationships: David discusses the impact of PR on his family life, particularly how his condition has prompted open conversations with his children about chronic illness. He values honesty and openness in relationships and believes that explaining PR to his family has strengthened their bond.

Message to Others: "PR may limit what my body can do on certain days, but it doesn't limit my outlook on life. Mindfulness has taught me to be present and to find joy in the small, simple moments. I've learned that I can still have a fulfilling life by adjusting my mindset."

These stories highlight the adaptability and resilience of PR patients who find unique ways to manage their symptoms, build supportive communities, and maintain positivity.

2. The Role of Caregivers

Caregivers play an essential role in the lives of PR patients, providing physical assistance, emotional support, and companionship. Their journey is one of dedication and compassion, and their perspectives offer insight into the challenges and rewards of caregiving for someone with PR.

Case Study 3: Maria's Story of Patience and Perseverance as a Caregiver

> Background: Maria's husband, Tom, was diagnosed with PR three years into their marriage. As his primary caregiver, Maria has seen firsthand how PR affects Tom's life, from the pain of flares to the fatigue and frustration that follows.
>
> Coping with Challenges: Maria describes the initial challenges of understanding PR and learning to adapt their daily routines around

Tom's symptoms. She struggled with feelings of helplessness, especially during intense flares when she could only offer comfort and encouragement.

Developing a Supportive Routine: Over time, Maria and Tom developed a system to manage PR together. They plan outings and activities around his symptom-free periods and keep essentials, like heating pads and comfortable seating, available at home. Maria finds comfort in connecting with other caregivers through support groups, where she can share her experiences and learn from others.

Message to Other Caregivers: "Caregiving for a loved one with PR is a journey of patience and flexibility. It's about finding joy in the moments you can share, even if they're small. The most valuable thing I've learned is that I can't take the pain away, but I can be there for him, and that's enough."

Case Study 4: James' Reflections as a Supportive
Friend

Background: James has been friends with
Eric, a PR patient, since high school. As Eric's
condition progressed, James became a
source of emotional support, helping Eric
navigate the social and emotional impacts
of living with PR.

Supporting from a Distance: While James
doesn't live with Eric, he makes a point of
checking in regularly, offering
encouragement and a listening ear. He
notes that one of the biggest ways he can
help is by validating Eric's experience and
being there without judgment.

Understanding PR as a Friend: James shares
that learning about PR has helped him
empathize with Eric's experiences,
recognizing that flares and limitations are
real, even if invisible. He has adapted his
expectations and finds ways to be flexible in
their plans, whether it means hanging out
at Eric's place or doing low-energy activities.

Message to Friends of PR Patients: "Being
there for a friend with PR doesn't mean you

need to fix anything; it's about showing up, listening, and being adaptable.

Understanding the unpredictability of PR has made our friendship stronger and deeper."

These caregiver perspectives underscore the importance of empathy, flexibility, and patience in supporting PR patients. Caregivers often learn to balance their own needs with those of their loved ones, finding meaning in the small ways they make a difference.

3. Family and Friends' Perspectives

PR affects more than just the individual diagnosed; it impacts family dynamics, friendships, and relationships. Family members and friends play a crucial role in supporting patients emotionally and practically. These perspectives offer a broader view of how PR influences relationships and the adjustments loved ones make to provide meaningful support.

Case Study 5: Anna's Journey as a Daughter

Background: Anna's mother, Emily, was diagnosed with PR when Anna was in college. The diagnosis brought them closer, as Anna became a primary support for her mother, who faced difficulties managing her daily tasks due to PR.

Supporting a Parent: Anna shares how she learned to help her mother without compromising her own independence. She balances her career and family life while making regular visits to help with errands and accompany her mother to medical appointments.

Lessons in Empathy: Anna explains that PR has taught her to be more empathetic and patient. Although she found it challenging to see her mother in pain, she realized the value of simply being present and offering her support.

Message to Family Members: "Living with a parent who has PR requires both patience and respect for their independence. My mom has shown incredible resilience, and I've learned to meet her where she is rather than trying to fix everything. Just being there and showing I care means the world to her."

Case Study 6: Carol's Experience as a Supportive Sibling

Background: Carol's younger sister, Lisa, was diagnosed with PR in her late 20s. As Lisa struggled with pain and fatigue, Carol became her confidante and often accompanied her to appointments and treatments.

Learning About PR Together: Carol shares how she and Lisa learned about PR together, researching symptoms, treatments, and support resources. Carol initially felt helpless, but over time, she found comfort in educating herself about PR so she could better support Lisa.

Strengthening Sibling Bond: The experience brought Carol and Lisa closer, helping them communicate more openly. Carol notes that their relationship has deepened, as Lisa feels more comfortable sharing her challenges without fear of judgment.

Message to Siblings: "Being there for a sibling with PR means more than just offering help—it's about understanding and empathy. I've learned that by showing compassion and being open to learning about her condition, I can make a real difference in her life."

These stories from family and friends illustrate the power of empathy, understanding, and adaptability in supporting loved ones with PR. Even when they cannot relieve the physical symptoms, their presence and support provide essential comfort and reassurance.

Summary

Patient and caregiver stories bring to life the experiences of those impacted by palindromic rheumatism, shedding light on the daily resilience required to navigate a life marked by unpredictability. Patients demonstrate adaptability and determination as they develop personalized coping strategies and find new ways to live fulfilling lives despite the limitations PR imposes. Caregivers, family, and friends also play a pivotal role, offering practical and emotional support, patience, and understanding that help PR patients feel validated and cared for.

Through these personal perspectives, we see the importance of community, empathy, and open communication in managing the challenges of PR. The strength and dedication of patients and their support networks underscore a central message: while PR is a difficult journey, it is one that can be navigated successfully with the right support, compassion, and resilience.

In the next chapter, we will explore the latest research and future directions in PR, looking at emerging treatments, ongoing studies, and potential advances that may offer new hope to those affected by this condition.

CHAPTER SEVEN:

RESEARCH AND FUTURE DIRECTIONS IN PALINDROMIC RHEUMATISM

The scientific understanding of palindromic rheumatism (PR) is continually evolving, as researchers work to uncover the mechanisms driving this unique, episodic form of arthritis. While PR is relatively rare and remains less studied compared to more prevalent conditions like rheumatoid arthritis (RA), recent advances in immunology, genetics, and biomarker research are beginning to shed light on this condition. These insights not only help us better understand PR but also pave the way for improved diagnostic methods, more targeted treatments, and potentially even preventative measures.

This chapter explores current research findings, promising therapeutic innovations, and future directions in PR research. These advances offer hope for improved quality of life and, ultimately, more personalized care for those affected by PR.

1. Current Research in PR

Recent research into PR has focused on understanding the immunological and genetic components of the disease. Although much of PR's pathology remains a mystery, these studies have provided valuable insights into the condition's underlying mechanisms.

Genetic and Immunological Insights:

Genetic Markers and Susceptibility: Studies suggest that PR may share certain genetic markers with RA and other autoimmune diseases, such as variations in the HLA-DRB1 gene. This gene, part of the major histocompatibility complex, plays a crucial role in immune system function and has been associated with a predisposition to autoimmune diseases. Although not all PR patients carry this genetic marker, its presence suggests that certain individuals may be genetically predisposed to developing PR.

Autoantibodies and Immune Response: Autoantibodies, such as rheumatoid factor (RF) and anti-cyclic citrullinated peptide (anti-CCP) antibodies, are commonly associated with RA and are also found in some PR patients. The presence of these antibodies indicates that the immune system may mistakenly attack the body's tissues, leading to episodic inflammation in the joints. The presence of anti-CCP antibodies, in particular, is linked to a higher likelihood of progressing from PR to RA, emphasizing the importance of monitoring PR patients for any changes in their condition.

Cytokines and Inflammatory Pathways:

Cytokines are signaling proteins that play a central role in the body's immune response. In PR, researchers have identified specific cytokines, such as interleukin-6 (IL-6) and tumor necrosis factor-alpha (TNF-α), which may be elevated during flares. These cytokines are associated with inflammation and are also key players in other autoimmune diseases.

Understanding the cytokine profile in PR patients provides valuable insights into potential therapeutic targets. Drugs that inhibit specific cytokines, like TNF-α inhibitors used in RA, may one day be adapted to treat PR if similar inflammatory pathways are found to drive the condition.

Role of Environmental Triggers:

Environmental factors, including infections, stress, and even hormonal changes, may trigger PR flares in genetically predisposed individuals. Some studies suggest that infections, particularly viral infections, might activate the immune response, setting off inflammatory episodes in the joints. This area of research is still developing, but understanding these triggers may help patients avoid flare-inducing factors and assist in developing preventive strategies.

These findings underscore the complex interplay of genetic, immunological, and environmental factors in PR. By continuing to study these areas, researchers hope to provide more specific diagnostic markers and improve patient outcomes through targeted therapies.

2. Emerging Treatments for PR

As researchers learn more about the mechanisms underlying PR, new treatment approaches are emerging. While conventional treatments like nonsteroidal anti-inflammatory drugs (NSAIDs) and disease-modifying antirheumatic drugs (DMARDs) remain the standard, there is a growing interest in more targeted therapies that could reduce flare frequency and severity.

Biologic Therapies:

> Biologic drugs are made from living cells and are designed to target specific components of the immune system. Commonly used in RA, biologics that target cytokines (such as TNF-α inhibitors and interleukin-6 inhibitors) are being explored for PR. These drugs work by blocking inflammatory pathways and may help reduce the frequency or intensity of flares in PR patients with persistent or severe symptoms.

> Examples of Biologics in Research: Drugs such as adalimumab, infliximab, and tocilizumab have shown effectiveness in RA

and are being tested for PR in certain cases. Initial studies suggest that some PR patients experience symptom relief with biologics, though further research is needed to establish long-term efficacy and safety specifically for PR.

JAK Inhibitors:

Janus kinase (JAK) inhibitors are another class of targeted therapies that modulate the immune response. By interfering with specific signaling pathways, JAK inhibitors help reduce inflammation at a cellular level. In RA, JAK inhibitors like tofacitinib and baricitinib have proven effective, and researchers are exploring their potential use in PR.

Advantages of JAK Inhibitors: These oral medications may offer a more convenient alternative to injectable biologics. If clinical trials confirm their effectiveness in PR, JAK inhibitors could provide a new option for patients who do not respond to traditional treatments.

Potential for Targeted DMARDs:

> Targeted DMARDs, such as hydroxychloroquine, are widely used in PR and have a favorable side effect profile compared to other immunosuppressive medications. Researchers are investigating additional DMARDs with targeted effects that could further reduce flares with minimal immune suppression.

> Ongoing Studies: Methotrexate, leflunomide, and sulfasalazine are among the DMARDs being studied to understand their long-term effects and efficacy in PR patients, particularly those with frequent or severe flares. As research continues, these drugs may be optimized for PR and refined based on specific patient needs.

These emerging treatments hold promise for offering PR patients more options and more effective symptom control. However, further clinical trials are needed to validate the efficacy and safety of these therapies in PR specifically.

3. Advances in Diagnostics

Current diagnostics for PR rely heavily on symptom patterns, laboratory markers, and the exclusion of other conditions. Researchers are working to refine diagnostic techniques, improve early detection, and identify biomarkers that may help distinguish PR from other types of arthritis or predict disease progression.

Biomarkers for Early Detection:

> Researchers are actively studying biomarkers that could enable earlier and more accurate PR diagnosis. Autoantibodies, inflammatory markers, and cytokine profiles are potential biomarkers that could be used to confirm PR in its early stages.

> Promising Biomarkers: Anti-CCP antibodies are one biomarker of interest, as they are present in both PR and RA. Researchers are exploring the use of these antibodies in combination with other markers, such as cytokines like IL-6, to create a diagnostic profile unique to PR.

Imaging Techniques:

Advances in imaging technology are enabling earlier detection of inflammation and joint changes in PR patients, even during periods of remission. Ultrasound and MRI remain valuable tools, and newer imaging techniques with higher sensitivity are being explored to capture subtle signs of inflammation that may not be visible on traditional X-rays.

Use of MRI in Monitoring PR: MRI can detect inflammation in soft tissues, such as tendons and ligaments, that are often involved in PR flares. By using MRI scans during both flare and remission periods, researchers hope to better understand the tissue-level effects of PR and identify early signs of disease progression.

Genetic Testing and Personalized Medicine:

Genetic testing may play a role in diagnosing PR or predicting disease course in the future. If specific genetic markers are confirmed to be associated with PR, genetic screening could help identify individuals at higher risk, potentially enabling preventive interventions.

Personalized Treatment Approaches: Genetic testing combined with biomarker analysis could allow for more personalized treatment approaches, tailoring medications to the individual's genetic profile and immune response. This precision medicine approach is still in its early stages but holds promise for providing more effective, targeted treatments for PR.

Advances in diagnostics could significantly reduce the time to diagnosis for PR patients, allowing for earlier intervention and potentially better outcomes.

4. Future Directions and Potential Cures

While there is no cure for PR, ongoing research may lead to new treatment approaches that provide more lasting remission or even preventative measures. Future research is focused on the following key areas:

Development of Preventative Therapies:

Understanding the environmental triggers and genetic predispositions associated with PR may one day allow researchers to develop preventative therapies. For instance, vaccines or immune-modulating drugs could potentially prevent PR in individuals identified as high-risk based on their genetic and immunological profiles.

Exploring Viral Triggers: Studies are investigating whether certain viruses play a role in triggering PR in genetically predisposed individuals. If specific viral triggers are confirmed, future research could explore antiviral therapies or vaccines as preventive measures for PR.

Stem Cell Therapy and Regenerative Medicine:

Stem cell therapy and regenerative medicine are promising fields that could one day provide innovative treatments for autoimmune diseases, including PR. Mesenchymal stem cells (MSCs), for example, have shown potential in reducing inflammation and repairing damaged tissues in other inflammatory conditions.

Application of Stem Cells in PR: While still experimental, stem cell therapies may offer PR patients a way to reduce inflammation without the need for long-term immune suppression. Clinical trials in RA and other forms of arthritis are exploring the feasibility of stem cell treatments, and similar trials in PR may follow.

Further Understanding of Disease Progression:

Not all PR patients progress to RA, but understanding the factors that influence this progression is critical. Research is focused on identifying which patients are at higher risk of developing RA and which factors—such as genetic markers, autoantibody levels, or inflammatory markers—may predict this transition.

Potential for Early Intervention: If researchers can reliably identify patients at risk of progression to RA, early interventions could be implemented to slow or prevent the transition. This approach is similar to preventive strategies used in individuals with early RA symptoms, where DMARDs or biologics are introduced early to prevent joint damage.

These future directions offer hope for new, more effective treatments for PR, with the potential for less invasive options, earlier interventions, and even preventive measures that could change the lives of PR patients.

Summary

Research into palindromic rheumatism is advancing, offering new insights into its genetic, immunological, and environmental triggers. Emerging therapies, such as biologics and JAK inhibitors, provide targeted treatment options, while advances in diagnostics may allow for earlier and more accurate detection of PR. As scientists continue to explore the mechanisms behind PR, new diagnostic tools and treatment options are on the horizon, providing hope for more personalized and effective care.

Although a cure remains elusive, the future of PR research is promising. Innovations in stem cell therapy, personalized medicine, and genetic testing could potentially reshape the landscape of PR treatment, providing patients with more control over their symptoms and improved quality of life. By supporting and following research efforts, PR patients and their caregivers can stay informed about breakthroughs that may one day transform the standard of care for this complex condition.

In the next chapter, we will discuss practical resources and support networks available for PR patients, including educational tools, advocacy organizations, and community groups that provide essential support in navigating life with PR.

CHAPTER EIGHT:

RESOURCES AND SUPPORT FOR PR PATIENTS

Living with palindromic rheumatism (PR) can be challenging, but the journey is made easier with the right resources and support networks. While PR is a rare and often misunderstood condition, there are organizations, educational tools, and communities dedicated to helping patients navigate the unique challenges it presents. Connecting with these resources not only provides practical assistance but also fosters a sense of community and shared understanding among those affected by PR.

In this chapter, we'll explore a variety of resources available to PR patients, including medical support, educational materials, online and in-person communities, and advocacy opportunities. These resources empower patients to better understand and manage their condition, build supportive relationships, and raise awareness of PR within their communities.

1. Finding Medical and Community Support

Medical and community support resources provide invaluable guidance for PR patients and their families. Whether through healthcare professionals, organizations, or community groups, these support systems help PR patients access accurate information, receive quality care, and find emotional support.

Rheumatology Clinics and Specialists:

> Consulting with a rheumatologist who has experience with autoimmune and inflammatory diseases is essential for PR patients. Rheumatology clinics are equipped to provide specialized care, diagnostic services, and tailored treatment plans. Some clinics also offer resources such as support groups or patient education programs.

> Finding the Right Specialist: The American College of Rheumatology and similar professional organizations offer directories of certified rheumatologists, which can help patients find a specialist in their area.

PR and Autoimmune Disease Organizations:

The Arthritis Foundation: The Arthritis Foundation offers resources and support for various types of arthritis, including PR. Their website provides educational materials, access to support groups, and information on clinical trials and new treatments.

National Institute of Arthritis and Musculoskeletal and Skin Diseases (NIAMS): Part of the National Institutes of Health, NIAMS provides in-depth information on PR, including treatment options and research updates. Their website is an excellent resource for patients who want to stay informed about advancements in PR care.

Rheumatoid Arthritis Support Organizations: Since PR shares some characteristics with RA, organizations that support RA patients may also offer helpful resources. Groups such as the Rheumatoid Arthritis Support Network (RASN) and the International Foundation for Autoimmune & Autoinflammatory Arthritis (AiArthritis) provide resources for people with similar symptoms and can often connect patients to PR-specific information.

Local Support Groups and Peer Networks:

Many communities have local support groups that provide a safe space for people with autoimmune diseases to share experiences, challenges, and coping strategies. While PR-specific groups may be limited, autoimmune support groups can offer insights and practical advice that are relevant to PR patients.

Benefits of Peer Networks: Peer networks allow PR patients to connect with others who understand their journey. These connections provide emotional support, reduce feelings of isolation, and enable patients to exchange tips on managing daily life with PR.

Connecting with these support resources can help PR patients build a network of professionals and peers who understand their condition, providing a foundation for effective management and emotional support.

2. Educational Resources

Understanding PR and staying informed about the latest research and treatments is essential for patients who want to take an active role in managing their condition. Educational resources, including books, online materials, and research publications, offer reliable information that empowers PR patients to make informed decisions about their care.

Books and Guides on PR and Autoimmune Conditions:

> "The Autoimmune Solution" by Dr. Amy Myers: This book provides insights into autoimmune diseases and discusses lifestyle strategies to manage symptoms, such as diet and stress reduction. While not specific to PR, it offers valuable guidance for reducing inflammation and enhancing immune health.

> "Anti-Inflammatory Eating for a Happy, Healthy Brain" by Michelle Babb: This book introduces readers to anti-inflammatory eating, with practical tips and recipes that

can benefit PR patients by reducing potential dietary triggers for inflammation.

PR-Specific Patient Guides: Some medical institutions or PR organizations publish guides that cover PR in detail. These guides provide an overview of symptoms, treatments, and lifestyle adjustments that may help manage the condition.

Research Publications and Journals:

Staying updated on current research can give patients and caregivers insight into new treatments and advancements in PR care. Websites like PubMed and ResearchGate provide access to studies on PR, though some articles may require institutional access.

Journal Recommendations: Journals like Arthritis Research & Therapy, The Journal of Rheumatology, and Annals of the Rheumatic Diseases frequently publish research on autoimmune diseases, including studies on PR. These journals provide the latest scientific findings and may include articles on emerging therapies or diagnostic tools.

Websites and Online Courses:

> Coursera and edX: These platforms offer courses on immunology, chronic disease management, and arthritis that may interest PR patients and caregivers seeking a deeper understanding of PR. Courses on inflammation and autoimmunity can provide insight into the mechanisms of PR.

> NIH and Mayo Clinic Websites: Both sites offer reliable, patient-friendly information on PR and related conditions. They cover a range of topics, from treatment options to lifestyle tips, and are regularly updated to reflect the latest medical guidelines.

Accessing these educational resources enables PR patients to expand their knowledge of the disease, empowering them to advocate for themselves and make informed choices in their treatment and lifestyle.

3. Online and In-Person Communities

Connecting with others who share similar experiences is invaluable for PR patients. Online and in-person communities provide spaces for sharing stories, asking questions, and exchanging tips. Through these communities, patients find camaraderie, understanding, and inspiration.

Online Forums and Social Media Groups:

> Reddit: Subreddits like r/autoimmune, r/rheumatoid, and r/ChronicIllness offer forums for patients with autoimmune conditions, including PR. Patients share their experiences, ask questions, and provide support to one another, fostering a sense of community online.

> Facebook Support Groups: There are several Facebook groups dedicated to PR and autoimmune conditions, such as "Palindromic Rheumatism Support" and "Autoimmune Warriors." These groups allow members to post questions, share updates, and connect with people who understand the day-to-day challenges of PR.

> The Mighty: The Mighty is an online community focused on chronic illness and mental health. Patients with PR and other chronic conditions share articles, advice,

and stories, creating a supportive environment for those navigating similar challenges.

Patient Advocacy Organizations:

Arthritis Foundation Virtual Events: The Arthritis Foundation hosts virtual events, such as webinars and live Q&A sessions, that provide opportunities for patients to learn from experts and connect with other patients. Topics range from managing flares to understanding new treatment options.

AiArthritis Voices 360: AiArthritis Voices 360 is a program that offers podcasts, virtual meetups, and panel discussions on autoimmune and autoinflammatory arthritis. These sessions feature expert speakers and patient advocates, making them an excellent resource for PR patients seeking both information and support.

In-Person Support Groups:

Local Arthritis Support Groups: Many cities and hospitals offer in-person support groups for arthritis and autoimmune disease patients. Although PR-specific groups are rare, general arthritis groups provide support and camaraderie among people facing similar struggles.

Community Centers and Health Organizations: Local community centers, libraries, and health organizations sometimes host support meetings for chronic illness and autoimmune conditions. These gatherings allow patients to connect face-to-face, share experiences, and learn from others in their community.

Whether connecting online or in person, these communities provide a safe space for PR patients to share their journey, ask questions, and build friendships that offer strength and understanding.

4. Advocacy and Raising Awareness

Advocacy plays a critical role in increasing awareness of PR and encouraging more research into the condition. By participating in advocacy efforts, PR patients and caregivers can contribute to better representation, more funding for research, and a stronger support network for the PR community.

Participating in Awareness Campaigns:

Arthritis Awareness Month: Observed in May, Arthritis Awareness Month is an opportunity to promote understanding and support for all forms of arthritis, including PR. Patients and caregivers can participate by sharing their stories on social media, organizing local events, or joining awareness walks.

World Autoimmune Arthritis Day: This global event, held annually on May 20th, aims to raise awareness about autoimmune forms of arthritis. Patients and supporters are encouraged to share information on social media and participate in virtual events to spread awareness about PR and related conditions.

Becoming a Patient Advocate:

Advocacy Training Programs: Programs offered by organizations like the Arthritis Foundation teach patients how to become effective advocates. These training sessions cover skills like communicating with legislators, raising public awareness, and educating healthcare providers on patient perspectives.

Speaking at Conferences and Events: Some PR patients choose to share their stories at medical conferences, panel discussions, and support group meetings. By speaking about their experiences, patients contribute to a greater understanding of PR, encouraging healthcare providers to recognize and address the unique challenges of the condition.

Supporting PR Research:

Donating to Research Initiatives: Supporting organizations that fund PR research, such as the Arthritis Foundation or the National Institute of Arthritis and Musculoskeletal and Skin Diseases, helps increase the resources available for studies into new treatments and diagnostic tools.

Participating in Clinical Trials: Some PR patients may qualify for clinical trials that explore new treatments or interventions. By participating in these studies, patients can contribute to scientific knowledge and help future PR patients access better care. Websites like ClinicalTrials.gov provide information on ongoing studies that accept PR patients.

Advocacy efforts help raise awareness of PR within both the medical community and the public, encouraging greater empathy, funding, and research into this rare condition. Every effort—big or small—contributes to building a stronger, more informed community.

Summary

Resources and support are essential for managing the complexities of palindromic rheumatism. Medical and community support networks provide the guidance and companionship needed for effective management, while educational resources empower PR patients to make informed decisions about their care. Online and in-person communities create spaces for connection and shared experiences, and advocacy efforts raise awareness of PR, fostering better understanding and encouraging more research.

By utilizing these resources, PR patients and caregivers can find support and inspiration while also playing an active role in building a brighter future for the PR community. Whether it's through participating in advocacy events, joining support groups, or staying informed about the latest research, PR patients have numerous ways to connect, learn, and contribute.

In the final chapter, we'll address frequently asked questions about PR, debunk common myths, and provide clarifications on topics that matter most to PR patients and their families.

CHAPTER NINE:

FAQS AND MYTH-BUSTING

Palindromic rheumatism (PR) is a unique and often misunderstood condition, which can lead to confusion and misconceptions for both patients and those around them. Given PR's episodic nature and its overlap with symptoms of other autoimmune diseases, patients frequently encounter myths and misunderstandings about their condition. This chapter aims to answer some of the most frequently asked questions about PR, providing accurate information and addressing common myths. By understanding the facts, PR patients and their loved ones can feel more confident in navigating the complexities of this condition.

1. Common Questions about PR

The following questions reflect the most common concerns that PR patients and caregivers encounter. Understanding these topics can clarify many aspects of PR, from diagnosis to treatment options.

Q1: Is PR the same as rheumatoid arthritis (RA)?

Answer: No, PR and RA are distinct conditions, though they share some similarities. PR is characterized by episodic flares of joint pain, swelling, and inflammation that completely resolve between episodes, leaving no permanent joint damage. RA, on the other hand, is a chronic, progressive condition that causes continuous inflammation and often leads to joint erosion and deformities over time. While some PR patients may eventually develop RA, many do not, and the two diseases have different courses and treatments.

Q2: Can PR be cured?

Answer: Currently, there is no cure for PR. However, treatment options can help manage symptoms, reduce flare frequency, and improve quality of life. Medications, lifestyle adjustments, and complementary therapies can make a significant difference in controlling the symptoms. Ongoing research offers hope for future advancements, but for now, PR is considered a chronic condition that can be managed rather than cured.

Q3: Is PR considered an autoimmune disease?

Answer: Yes, PR is generally classified as an autoimmune condition. In autoimmune diseases, the immune system mistakenly attacks healthy tissues, leading to inflammation and symptoms like joint pain. The exact mechanisms of PR are not fully understood, but studies suggest that immune dysregulation plays a central role in causing flares.

Q4: How does PR affect daily life?

Answer: PR affects each person differently. Some individuals experience infrequent, mild flares, while others may have more severe and frequent episodes that interfere with daily activities. PR's unpredictability can make it challenging to plan or commit to activities, and patients may need to adapt their schedules, incorporate rest periods, or use assistive devices during flares. Emotional resilience and a strong support network are essential for managing the impact of PR on daily life.

Q5: Can lifestyle changes help manage PR symptoms?

Answer: Yes, lifestyle changes can play an important role in managing PR. Anti-inflammatory diets, regular low-impact exercise, stress reduction techniques, and adequate sleep have all been shown to support overall health and may help reduce flare frequency or severity. However, lifestyle changes should be viewed as a complement to medical treatment rather than a replacement, as PR requires a holistic approach for optimal management.

Q6: Is PR a hereditary condition?

Answer: PR is not considered directly hereditary, but genetic factors may increase an individual's susceptibility. Certain genetic markers associated with autoimmune diseases, such as variations in the HLA-DRB1 gene, have been found in some PR patients. Having a family history of autoimmune diseases may slightly increase the risk of developing PR, though the condition is influenced by a combination of genetic and environmental factors.

Q7: Are there any warning signs that a PR flare is coming?

Answer: Some patients report subtle signs that a flare is about to occur, such as mild joint stiffness, fatigue, or a general feeling of malaise. However, many PR flares begin without warning. Keeping a symptom diary may help some patients identify personal triggers or patterns, but the episodic and unpredictable nature of PR makes it challenging to anticipate flares with certainty.

Q8: Is PR associated with other health risks?

Answer: PR is primarily limited to joint inflammation and does not typically involve systemic issues. However, because PR shares some characteristics with other autoimmune conditions, PR patients are slightly more likely to develop other autoimmune diseases, such as RA or lupus. Regular check-ups and close monitoring with a rheumatologist can help manage PR and detect any changes in health.

These FAQs provide a foundation for understanding PR and address many of the uncertainties patients face. By clearing up these common questions, patients and caregivers can feel better equipped to manage PR.

2. Debunking Myths about Palindromic Rheumatism

Misconceptions about PR can lead to unnecessary stress and confusion for patients. By debunking these myths, we aim to provide clarity and encourage a more informed understanding of the condition.

Myth 1: "PR is just mild rheumatoid arthritis."

> Reality: While PR and RA share some symptoms, they are distinct conditions. PR is episodic, meaning flares come and go, often with complete symptom relief between episodes. RA, on the other hand, is a chronic, progressive condition that leads to permanent joint damage over time. Not all PR patients develop RA, and PR has a unique disease course that differs significantly from RA.

Myth 2: "PR doesn't need treatment because it doesn't cause permanent damage."

> Reality: Although PR typically does not cause joint damage, untreated flares can still cause significant pain, discomfort, and a reduced quality of life. Managing PR with appropriate treatments can reduce flare frequency and intensity, helping patients maintain mobility and improve their day-to-

day functioning. Additionally, some PR patients may progress to RA, so regular monitoring and treatment are essential.

Myth 3: "Only older people get PR."

Reality: PR can affect individuals of all ages, including young adults and, in rare cases, children. While the exact age of onset varies, PR is most commonly diagnosed in adults between their 20s and 50s. The misconception that PR only affects older people may delay diagnosis for younger patients who do not fit the traditional profile of arthritis patients.

Myth 4: "PR symptoms are all in your head."

Reality: PR is a real, medically recognized condition that causes episodic joint inflammation, pain, and swelling. Just because symptoms disappear between flares does not make them any less real or less serious. The lack of visible symptoms between flares can lead to misunderstandings, but PR's impact on patients' lives is genuine, and the condition requires proper medical management.

Myth 5: "PR will inevitably progress to rheumatoid arthritis."

Reality: While some PR patients do eventually develop RA, many do not. Studies indicate that about one-third of PR patients progress to RA, often within five years of diagnosis, but two-thirds remain with PR as a distinct condition. Monitoring by a rheumatologist is important to track any changes, but progression is not guaranteed.

Myth 6: "People with PR shouldn't exercise."

Reality: Exercise can be beneficial for people with PR, helping maintain joint mobility, strengthen muscles, and improve overall health. Low-impact activities, such as swimming, walking, and yoga, are often well-suited to PR patients. However, it is important to listen to the body and avoid overexertion during flares. An exercise plan tailored to individual needs, ideally created with the guidance of a healthcare provider or physical therapist, can support joint health without triggering flares.

Myth 7: "PR is not serious because it's episodic."

Reality: PR's episodic nature can create the impression that it is less serious than chronic conditions. However, PR can significantly impact quality of life, causing severe pain, emotional stress, and limitations on daily activities. The unpredictability of flares adds an additional layer of complexity, as patients cannot predict when symptoms will strike. Proper management and support are crucial for maintaining a good quality of life with PR.

Dispelling these myths about PR allows patients to have more accurate expectations and understanding of their condition. It also encourages empathy from friends, family, and healthcare providers who may not fully grasp the challenges PR patients face.

Summary

Palindromic rheumatism is a complex, often misunderstood condition. By addressing frequently asked questions and debunking common myths, we hope to provide patients and caregivers with a clearer understanding of PR. Knowing the facts about PR helps patients advocate for themselves and ensures they receive the proper support and treatment.

Through this chapter, we have clarified essential aspects of PR, from diagnosis to daily life challenges, and addressed misunderstandings that can create barriers to care and support. By fostering a more accurate perception of PR, patients can feel more empowered and confident in managing their condition.

As this book concludes, our hope is that PR patients, caregivers, and healthcare providers alike have gained a deeper understanding of this rare condition. Equipped with knowledge, support, and practical strategies, individuals affected by PR can navigate their journey with resilience, self-compassion, and a sense of community.

CONCLUSION:

MOVING FORWARD WITH PR

Living with palindromic rheumatism (PR) is a journey marked by unpredictability, resilience, and adaptability. From the initial onset of symptoms to the challenges of diagnosis, treatment, and daily management, each step can feel like a new hurdle to overcome. Yet, as this book has shown, PR patients are not alone in their experiences. By understanding the nature of PR, exploring effective treatments, and connecting with supportive communities, individuals affected by PR can build a path forward that brings both relief and resilience.

As we conclude, let us reflect on some of the key insights and takeaways from this journey through PR, with a hopeful look toward the future for all those impacted by this condition.

The Power of Understanding and Advocacy

One of the most significant barriers to effective management of PR is a lack of awareness and understanding—both for patients and within the broader medical community. Given PR's rarity and episodic nature, it's not uncommon for patients to encounter misunderstandings or even skepticism about their symptoms. Yet, with knowledge comes empowerment. By understanding PR's characteristics, common treatment options, and effective management strategies, patients are better equipped to advocate for their needs, communicate clearly with healthcare providers, and make informed decisions about their care.

For friends, family, and caregivers, learning about PR fosters greater empathy and understanding. Recognizing that PR is a medically recognized, legitimate condition—even though it is episodic and doesn't always leave physical evidence— allows loved ones to offer the compassion and support that PR patients need, whether they are experiencing a flare or feeling well.

Community and Connection

One of the most powerful forms of support for PR patients is connecting with others who share similar experiences. Throughout this book, we've seen the value of patient stories and peer support in providing comfort, validation, and practical advice. Online forums, support groups, and social media communities create spaces where PR patients can share their stories, ask questions, and learn from one another. These communities remind patients that they are not alone on this journey and that others understand the unique challenges they face.

Family members, friends, and caregivers are also an integral part of the support system. The understanding and patience of loved ones can make a world of difference, helping PR patients maintain a sense of normalcy and positivity, even during difficult flares. By creating a network of support, PR patients find strength in relationships that reinforce their resilience.

Adapting to Life with PR

Living with PR requires a blend of adaptability, patience, and proactive self-care. By incorporating lifestyle adjustments—such as adopting anti-inflammatory diets, engaging in gentle exercise, prioritizing sleep, and practicing stress management—PR patients can improve their quality of life and potentially reduce the frequency or severity of flares. These adjustments support not only physical well-being but also mental and emotional health, which are crucial in managing the stresses of living with a chronic condition.

Through careful planning, pacing, and communicating needs openly, PR patients can find ways to continue engaging in activities they love, maintaining work responsibilities, and nurturing personal relationships. While life with PR may require adaptations, it does not have to prevent a fulfilling, active, and meaningful life.

Hope for the Future

Research in PR is still in its early stages, but progress is being made. Advances in understanding genetic and immunological factors, as well as the development of targeted therapies, offer hope that more effective treatments will become available. The potential for biologics, JAK inhibitors, and even future regenerative therapies could transform the standard of care for PR, providing patients with more options for relief and improving their quality of life. New diagnostic tools, such as biomarkers and advanced imaging techniques, may also enable earlier detection and more accurate diagnoses, helping patients access effective treatment sooner.

As research progresses, the PR community plays a vital role in advocating for continued studies and funding. Each patient story, each advocacy effort, and each participation in a clinical trial brings us one step closer to better understanding and ultimately improving life for everyone affected by PR.

A Message of Resilience and Hope

Living with PR is not easy, and it's natural for patients to feel frustrated or discouraged at times. Yet, as we have seen throughout this book, PR patients are strong, resilient, and resourceful. They face each day with courage, adapting to the challenges that arise with creativity, humor, and determination. By embracing the strategies and resources available, PR patients can continue to build a life that aligns with their values and brings them joy, despite the limitations of the condition.

To every PR patient reading this book, know that your journey is unique, and your resilience is inspiring. Remember that while PR is part of your life, it does not define who you are or what you can accomplish. With the support of your community, healthcare providers, and loved ones, you have the strength to face each flare, navigate each uncertainty, and live fully within the parameters of your condition.

As we conclude, let this message serve as a reminder that living with PR is a journey marked by resilience, hope, and the unwavering determination to thrive. Though the path may not always be easy, it is one that can be traveled with courage and compassion.

With knowledge, support, and a spirit of perseverance, PR patients can look forward to a future filled with hope and possibility.

APPENDIX 1:

GLOSSARY OF TERMS

Antibody

A protein produced by the immune system in response to the presence of a foreign substance (antigen). Antibodies bind to specific antigens to help neutralize or eliminate them. In autoimmune diseases, autoantibodies may mistakenly target the body's own tissues.

Anti-Cyclic Citrullinated Peptide (Anti-CCP)

An antibody that targets proteins in the body that contain a specific type of modification, called citrullination. Anti-CCP is commonly found in rheumatoid arthritis (RA) patients and may also be present in some PR patients, helping to predict potential progression to RA.

Antinuclear Antibodies (ANA)

Antibodies that target the nucleus of cells. ANA tests are commonly used to diagnose autoimmune diseases, such as lupus. A positive ANA test can indicate an autoimmune response, though it is not specific to any one condition.

Autoimmune Disease

A condition in which the immune system mistakenly attacks the body's own cells, tissues, or organs, causing inflammation and damage. Examples include rheumatoid arthritis, lupus, and PR.

Biologic Therapy

A type of treatment derived from living organisms, usually proteins or antibodies, that specifically target certain parts of the immune system. Biologics are used to treat autoimmune diseases by reducing inflammation or altering immune system function.

C-Reactive Protein (CRP)

A protein produced by the liver in response to inflammation. Elevated CRP levels can indicate inflammation in the body, which is common in autoimmune conditions like PR during flares.

Chronic Condition

A long-lasting health condition that may not have a cure but can be managed with treatment. Chronic conditions, such as arthritis or diabetes, often require ongoing medical care.

Cytokines

Small proteins released by cells that play a key role in immune responses. Cytokines, such as interleukin-6 (IL-6) and tumor necrosis factor-alpha (TNF-α), are involved in inflammation and are often elevated in autoimmune diseases.

Disease-Modifying Antirheumatic Drugs (DMARDs)

A class of medications used to slow the progression of autoimmune diseases by targeting inflammation. Common DMARDs include methotrexate and hydroxychloroquine.

Erythrocyte Sedimentation Rate (ESR)

A blood test that measures the rate at which red blood cells settle in a test tube over a specified period. An elevated ESR indicates inflammation, often seen in autoimmune conditions like PR.

Flare

A sudden episode of increased symptoms or disease activity, such as pain, swelling, and inflammation in PR. Flares are temporary and may last from hours to days, with periods of relief in between.

HLA-DRB1

A gene that plays a role in immune system function and has been associated with a higher risk of developing autoimmune diseases. Specific variations in this gene are sometimes found in people with PR and RA.

Hydroxychloroquine

A DMARD commonly used to treat PR and other autoimmune conditions. Hydroxychloroquine reduces inflammation and is generally well-tolerated, making it a popular option for long-term management of PR.

Immunology

The branch of medicine that studies the immune system, its functions, and related diseases. Immunology research is key to understanding autoimmune conditions like PR.

Interleukin-6 (IL-6)

A cytokine that plays a major role in inflammation and is elevated in many autoimmune diseases. Targeting IL-6 can help reduce inflammation in diseases like RA and may also have potential in PR treatment.

Janus Kinase (JAK) Inhibitors

A class of medications that block the activity of certain enzymes involved in immune cell signaling. JAK inhibitors are used to reduce inflammation and are being explored as a treatment option for autoimmune diseases, including PR.

Joint Erosion

Damage to the bone and cartilage in joints, often seen in chronic conditions like RA. PR, by contrast, does not usually cause permanent joint damage, as symptoms resolve between flares.

Mesenchymal Stem Cells (MSCs)

A type of stem cell with anti-inflammatory properties, found in bone marrow, fat tissue, and other areas. MSC therapy is being researched as a potential treatment for autoimmune diseases, with the goal of reducing inflammation and promoting tissue repair.

Nonsteroidal Anti-Inflammatory Drugs (NSAIDs)

A class of medications used to relieve pain and reduce inflammation. NSAIDs, such as ibuprofen and naproxen, are commonly used by PR patients to manage pain during flares.

Palindromic Rheumatism (PR)

An episodic form of inflammatory arthritis characterized by sudden flares of joint pain, swelling, and inflammation that resolve completely between episodes. PR is considered an autoimmune disease and shares some features with RA, though it does not cause permanent joint damage.

Progression

The development or advancement of a disease over time. In PR, progression may refer to the potential for some patients to develop RA, although many patients do not experience this shift.

Rheumatoid Arthritis (RA)

A chronic, progressive autoimmune disease characterized by persistent inflammation in the joints, leading to joint erosion and deformity. RA shares some features with PR, but it has a different disease course and often causes permanent joint damage.

Rheumatoid Factor (RF)

An autoantibody commonly found in RA patients and sometimes present in PR patients. A positive RF test can indicate an autoimmune process but is not specific to PR or RA alone.

Symptom-Free Period

The time between PR flares when a patient experiences no symptoms. Symptom-free periods can vary widely in duration from person to person.

Tumor Necrosis Factor-Alpha (TNF-α)

A cytokine involved in systemic inflammation. TNF-α is a target of some biologic treatments for autoimmune diseases, as blocking its activity can reduce inflammation in conditions like RA.

Ultrasound

An imaging technique that uses sound waves to create images of structures within the body. In PR, ultrasound can help detect joint inflammation during a flare, even when there are no visible symptoms.

X-Ray

A standard imaging technique often used to assess joint health. In PR, X-rays are typically normal, as the condition does not cause lasting joint damage, unlike chronic conditions such as RA.

APPENDIX 2:

RESOURCES FOR PR PATIENTS AND CAREGIVERS

Navigating life with palindromic rheumatism (PR) can be challenging, but many resources are available to support patients, caregivers, and family members. From educational tools to support networks and advocacy organizations, these resources can provide guidance, community, and practical assistance. This appendix compiles some of the most valuable resources for understanding, managing, and coping with PR.

1. Educational and Medical Resources

Arthritis Foundation

> Website: [arthritis.org] (https://www.arthritis.org)

> Description: The Arthritis Foundation provides comprehensive resources on arthritis-related conditions, including PR. The site offers information on treatment, research updates, and ways to manage pain

and flares. It also includes support options, such as online and local community groups.

National Institute of Arthritis and Musculoskeletal and Skin Diseases (NIAMS)

Website: [niams.nih.gov] (https://www.niams.nih.gov)

Description: Part of the National Institutes of Health, NIAMS offers reliable, up-to-date information on PR and related autoimmune conditions. The site includes resources on current research, clinical trials, and general health guidance for managing musculoskeletal diseases.

Mayo Clinic

Website: [mayoclinic.org] (https://www.mayoclinic.org)

Description: Mayo Clinic provides detailed information on PR, symptoms, and treatment options. The website includes insights from medical professionals and offers additional resources for understanding and managing autoimmune diseases.

American College of Rheumatology (ACR)

Website: [rheumatology.org] (https://www.rheumatology.org)

Description: The ACR offers a "Find a Rheumatologist" tool to help patients connect with specialists. It also provides educational resources about rheumatic diseases, including PR, and publishes research updates and treatment guidelines for rheumatologists.

PubMed and ResearchGate

Websites: [pubmed.ncbi.nlm.nih.gov] (https://pubmed.ncbi.nlm.nih.gov) | [researchgate.net](https://www.researchgat e.net)

Description: These platforms provide access to medical research articles, including studies on PR, its treatments, and autoimmune mechanisms. While some articles may require institutional access, both sites offer a wealth of peer-reviewed information for those interested in the latest research.

2. Online Communities and Support Groups

Reddit - r/autoimmune and r/rheumatoid

Website: [reddit.com/r/autoimmune](https://www.reddit.com/r/autoimmune) | [reddit.com/r/rheumatoid](https://www.reddit.com/r/rheumatoid)

Description: These subreddits provide an online space where PR patients and those with autoimmune diseases share experiences, tips, and support. These forums are valuable for connecting with others who understand the challenges of PR.

The Mighty

Website: [themighty.com]
(https://www.themighty.com)

Description: The Mighty offers articles,
stories, and forums for people with chronic
illnesses and disabilities, including PR. Users
can join groups, participate in discussions,
and read personal stories shared by other
PR patients.

Facebook Groups - "Palindromic Rheumatism
Support" and "Autoimmune Warriors"

Website: Facebook (Search for groups by
name)

Description: Facebook hosts several support
groups dedicated to PR and autoimmune
diseases. These groups provide a platform
for sharing experiences, asking questions,
and finding encouragement from others
with PR.

Arthritis Foundation's Live Yes! Network

Website: [arthritis.org/liveyes] (https://www.arthritis.org/liveyes)

Description: The Live Yes! Network connects arthritis patients to online and local support groups. The platform includes forums for discussions on lifestyle, treatments, and coping strategies for people with PR and other forms of arthritis.

3. Tools and Apps for Symptom Tracking and Management

My Arthritis

Website/App: Available in app stores for iOS and Android

Description: My Arthritis is a mobile app that helps arthritis patients, including those with PR, track symptoms, manage medications, and monitor pain levels over time. The app generates reports that can be shared with healthcare providers.

CreakyJoints ArthritisPower

> Website: [arthritispower.org]
> (https://www.arthritispower.org)

> Description: ArthritisPower is a patient-centered research registry and app that allows users to track PR symptoms, medication usage, and other health data. It also connects patients with ongoing research opportunities to help advance arthritis care.

Flaredown

> Website/App: Available in app stores for iOS and Android

> Description: Flaredown is a mobile app designed for people with chronic illnesses to track their symptoms, medications, and potential triggers. PR patients can use it to monitor flare-ups and identify patterns that help inform treatment adjustments.

Symple Symptom Tracker

Website/App: Available in app stores for iOS and Android

Description: Symple is a customizable symptom-tracking app that allows users to record pain levels, emotional health, and other factors influencing well-being. The app enables PR patients to log daily health details, which can be shared with healthcare providers.

4. Advocacy and Awareness Organizations

International Foundation for Autoimmune & Autoinflammatory Arthritis (AiArthritis)

Website: [aiarthritis.org] (https://www.aiarthritis.org)

Description: AiArthritis is an advocacy organization focused on education, support, and research for autoimmune and autoinflammatory arthritis. The organization hosts awareness campaigns and educational webinars, providing PR patients with ways to participate in advocacy and connect with others in the autoimmune community.

Global Healthy Living Foundation (GHLF)

Website: [ghlf.org](https://www.ghlf.org)

Description: GHLF advocates for people with chronic diseases, including PR. The organization promotes patient education, access to healthcare, and support for individuals living with chronic pain. It offers free resources, newsletters, and events to keep patients informed and engaged.

National Organization for Rare Disorders (NORD)

Website: [rarediseases.org](https://www.rarediseases.org)

Description: NORD supports patients with rare diseases, including PR. They offer resources for patients and families, advocacy tools, and connections to clinical trials. NORD also provides a Rare Disease

Database that features information on PR and similar conditions.

World Autoimmune and Autoinflammatory Arthritis Day (WAAD)

Website: [autoimmunearthritisday.org] (https://www.autoimmunearthritisday.org)

Description: WAAD is an annual awareness event on May 20th focused on autoimmune and autoinflammatory arthritis conditions. PR patients and supporters are encouraged to participate in social media campaigns, virtual events, and advocacy activities to raise awareness and educate the public.

5. Clinical Trials and Research Participation

ClinicalTrials.gov

Website: [clinicaltrials.gov] (https://www.clinicaltrials.gov)

Description: This government-run database lists ongoing clinical trials worldwide. Patients with PR can search for clinical trials related to autoimmune diseases, arthritis, and emerging treatments, offering an opportunity to contribute to scientific research.

CenterWatch

Website: [centerwatch.com] (https://www.centerwatch.com)

Description: CenterWatch is a resource for patients interested in participating in clinical trials. The site includes information on clinical trial locations, eligibility criteria, and current studies on PR and other autoimmune diseases.

Arthritis Foundation's Clinical Trial Finder

Website: [arthritis.org/research/clinical-trials](https://www.arthritis.org/research/clinical-trials)

Description: This tool connects arthritis patients to clinical trials relevant to their condition, including PR. The Clinical Trial Finder helps users locate studies in their area and provides information on new treatments under investigation.

These resources serve as valuable tools for PR patients and caregivers, offering a combination of educational materials, community support, tracking tools, advocacy opportunities, and research participation. By accessing these resources, patients and caregivers can stay informed, connect with others, and take an active role in managing and understanding palindromic rheumatism.

Together, these organizations, tools, and communities create a network of support, helping PR patients and their loved ones navigate the challenges of this unique condition with knowledge, resilience, and hope.

BIBLIOGRAPHY

Books and Journals

1. Firestein, G. S., & Budd, R. C. (Eds.).

   Kelley's Textbook of Rheumatology (10th ed.). Elsevier, 2017.

   > Comprehensive reference on rheumatic diseases, including PR and autoimmune conditions.

2. Hochberg, M. C., Silman, A. J., Smolen, J. S., et al. (Eds.).

   Rheumatology (7th ed.). Elsevier, 2018.

   > Key resource for understanding the pathology and treatment of rheumatic diseases.

3. Arthritis Foundation.

   Your Personal Guide to Living Well with Arthritis. Arthritis Foundation, 2020.

Patient-focused guide offering lifestyle tips and treatment insights for arthritis-related conditions.

4. Myers, A. (2015).

The Autoimmune Solution: Prevent and Reverse the Full Spectrum of Inflammatory Symptoms and Diseases. Harper Wave.

Practical advice on diet and lifestyle adjustments for managing autoimmune diseases.

5. Terkeltaub, R. (2018).

Gout & Other Crystal Arthropathies. Elsevier.

Covers gout and differential diagnoses relevant to PR.

6. Arthritis Foundation.

[arthritis.org](https://www.arthritis.org)

> Educational resources on PR, treatment options, and patient advocacy opportunities.

7. National Institute of Arthritis and Musculoskeletal and Skin Diseases (NIAMS).

[niams.nih.gov](https://www.niams.nih.gov)

> Reliable medical information on PR, autoimmune conditions, and ongoing research.

8. American College of Rheumatology.

[rheumatology.org](https://www.rheumatology.org)

> Resources for patients and professionals, including treatment guidelines for rheumatic diseases.

9. Mayo Clinic.

[mayoclinic.org](https://www.mayoclinic.org)

   Comprehensive medical information on PR symptoms, diagnosis, and treatments.

10. The Mighty.

[themighty.com](https://www.themighty.com)

   Online community platform for chronic illness patients, including PR support groups and stories.

11. ClinicalTrials.gov.

[clinicaltrials.gov](https://www.clinicaltrials.gov)

   Database of ongoing clinical trials for PR and autoimmune diseases.

12. Reddit Communities.

[reddit.com/r/autoimmune](https://www.reddit.com/r/autoimmune)

Patient-driven discussions and shared experiences about PR and other autoimmune diseases.

13. CreakyJoints ArthritisPower.

[arthritispower.org] (https://www.arthritispower.org)

Tools for tracking symptoms and accessing research opportunities for arthritis patients.

14. Global Healthy Living Foundation (GHLF).

[ghlf.org](https://www.ghlf.org)

Advocacy and education for chronic disease patients, including those with PR.

Research Articles

15. Alarcón-Segovia, D., Díaz-Jouanen, E., & Coutiño, M. (1974).

"Palindromic Rheumatism: A Clinical Study of 146 Patients." The Journal of Rheumatology, 1(2), 146-155.

Foundational study on the clinical characteristics of PR.

16. Mattingly, P. C. (1987).

"Palindromic Rheumatism: Relationship to Rheumatoid Arthritis." Seminars in Arthritis and Rheumatism, 16(4), 206-215.

Explores the connection between PR and RA.

17. Quinn, M. A., Green, M. J., & Conaghan, P. G. (2001).

"Early Prediction of Rheumatoid Arthritis in Patients with Palindromic Rheumatism." Annals of the Rheumatic Diseases, 60(1), 31-36.

Focuses on the risk of progression from PR to RA.

18. Smolen, J. S., & Aletaha, D. (2018).

"Targets of Therapy for Rheumatoid Arthritis." New England Journal of Medicine, 379(8), 750-762.

Discusses therapeutic approaches relevant to autoimmune arthritis.

19. van Venrooij, W. J., van Beers, J. J. B. C., & Pruijn, G. J. M. (2011).

"Anti-CCP Antibodies: The Past, the Present, and the Future." Nature Reviews Rheumatology, 7(7), 391-398.

Review of anti-CCP antibodies in autoimmune conditions, including PR.

Advocacy and Support Organizations

20. International Foundation for Autoimmune &
Autoinflammatory Arthritis (AiArthritis).

[aiarthritis.org](https://www.aiarthritis.org)

Advocacy and resources for patients with
autoimmune and autoinflammatory arthritis
conditions.

21. National Organization for Rare Disorders
(NORD).

[rarediseases.org](https://www.rarediseases.org)

Information and resources for patients with
rare diseases, including PR.

22. World Autoimmune and Autoinflammatory
Arthritis Day (WAAD).

[autoimmunearthritisday.org](https://www.autoi
mmunearthritisday.org)

Annual awareness campaign focused on
autoimmune arthritis conditions.

www.ingramcontent.com/pod-product-compliance
Lightning Source LLC
Chambersburg PA
CBHW071459220526
45472CB00003B/862

9 7 9 8 3 0 0 5 6 1 9 9 4